Step by

Cross-sectional
Anatomy

Step by Step
Cross-sectional Anatomy

D Karthikeyan DMRD DNB
Chief Radiologist
Division of Computed Tomography and Body Imaging
Department of Imaging Sciences
KG Hospital and Postgraduate Institute
Coimbatore
Programme Director, Radeducation Pvt. Ltd.
Coimbatore

Deepa Chegu
Consultant Radiologist
GEM Hospital (P) Ltd
Coimbatore

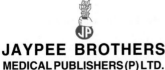

JAYPEE BROTHERS
MEDICAL PUBLISHERS (P) LTD.
New Delhi

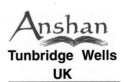

Tunbridge Wells
UK

First published in the UK by

Anshan Ltd
in 2006
6 Newlands Road
Tunbridge Wells
Kent TN4 9AT, UK

Tel/Fax: +44 (0)1892 557767
E-mail: info@anshan.co.uk
www.anshan.co.uk

ISBN-10 1 904798 80 2
ISBN-13 978 1 904798 80 4

British Library Cataloguing in Publication Data
A catalogue record for this book is available from the British Library

Printed in India by Paras Offset Pvt. Ltd., Naraina, New Delhi.

Preface

Computed tomography has changed the way of looking at the human anatomy dramatically. Knowledge and understanding of cross-sectional anatomy is essential for all those involved in performing CT scans. Designed for easy reference this illustrated manual is a practical first step guide towards interpretation of CT studies.

D Karthikeyan
Deepa Chegu

Contents

Contents

Chapter 1

Brain

BRAIN—AN OVERVIEW

Structure	Description	Significance
Forebrain	Prosencephalon	Comprised of: telencephalon or cerebral hemispheres and diencephalon; site of termination of cranial nerves I and II; contains lateral and third ventricles
Midbrain	Mesencephalon	Connects forebrain and hindbrain; site of origin of cranial nerves III and IV; contains cerebral aqueduct
Hindbrain	Rhombencephalon	Comprised of: metencephalon or pons and cerebellum and myelencephalon or medulla oblongata; site of origin for cranial nerves V-XII (except spinal part of accessory nerve); contains fourth ventricle
Telencephalon	Rostral part of forebrain	Comprised of: cerebral hemispheres and basal ganglia; contains lateral ventricles
Diencephalon	Caudal portion of forebrain	Comprised of: thalamus, metathalamus, subthalamus, epithalamus; contains third ventricle
Mesencephalon	Midbrain	Contains the corpora quadrigemina
Metencephalon	Rostral part of rhombencephalon	Comprised of: pons and cerebellum
Myelencephalon	Caudal part of rhombencephalon	Comprised of: medulla oblongata; medulla becomes continuous with the spinal cord at the level of the foramen magnum

FEATURES OF THE BRAIN—LATERAL VIEW

Structure	Description	Significance
Cerebral hemispheres	Telencephalon	Comprised of: cortex featuring gyri, sulci, fissures and lobes; commissures connecting parts; basal ganglia; contains lateral ventricles; termination of the olfactory tract
Longitudinal fissure	Midline, sagittal cleft separating the paired cerebral hemispheres	Contains the falx cerebri
Frontal pole	The most anterior part of the cerebral hemisphere	Frontal pole is part of the frontal lobe
Temporal pole	The most anterior part of the temporal lobe	
Occipital pole	The most posterior part of the cerebral hemisphere	Occipital pole is part of the occipital lobe; composed of primary visual cortex
Central sulcus	Separates frontal and parietal lobes	Separates the precentral gyrus (motor) from the postcentral gyrus (sensory)
Frontal lobe	Rostral to central sulcus	Contains prefrontal (emotions, personality) and precentral (primary and secondary motor) areas

Contd...

Contd...

Parietal lobe	Separated from the frontal lobe by the central sulcus, separated from occipital lobe by line through parieto-occipital sulcus	Contains the primary and secondary somatosensory areas
Temporal lobe	Separated from the frontal lobe by the lateral sulcus	Primarily concerned with hearing and memory/learning
Occipital lobe	Posterior to an imaginary line through parieto-occipital sulcus	Contains the primary and secondary visual cortex
Precentral gyrus	Most caudal gyrus of the frontal lobe; it lies rostral to the central sulcus	Contains the primary motor cortex
Postcentral gyrus	Most rostral gyrus of the parietal lobe; it lies caudal to the central sulcus	Contains the primary sensory cortex
Superior temporal gyrus	Gyrus between the lateral sulcus and the superior temporal sulcus	Contains the primary auditory cortex
Middle temporal gyrus	Gyrus between the superior and inferior temporal sulci	
Inferior temporal gyrus	Gyrus between the inferior temporal sulcus and the inferior margin of the temporal lobe	
Insula	Portion of the cerebrum located deeply within the lateral sulcus	Also known as the island of Reil
Straight gyrus	Gyrus located on the medial side of the olfactory tract	Also known as: gyrus rectus

Contd...

Contd...

Uncus	Portion of the cerebral cortex on the medial side of the parahippocampal gyrus and overlying the amygdala; located near the free edge of the tentorium cerebelli	Contains olfactory cortex
Longitudinal sulcus	Midline, sagittal cleft separating the paired cerebral hemispheres	Also known as: longitudinal fissure
Precentral sulcus	The sulcus anterior to the precentral gyrus	In conjunction with the central sulcus, it defines the precentral gyrus (motor)
Postcentral sulcus	The sulcus posterior to the postcentral gyrus	In conjunction with the central sulcus, it defines the postcentral gyrus (sensory)
Lateral sulcus	Separates frontal lobe and temporal lobe	The insula lies in the floor of this sulcus
Superior temporal sulcus	Sulcus between the superior and middle temporal gyri	Used to define the superior and middle temproal gyri
Inferior temporal sulcus	Sulcus between thle middle and inferior temporal gyri	Used to define the middle and inferior temporal gyri
Parieto-occipital sulcus	Sulcus between the parietal and occipital lobes	Landmark used to define the borders of the parietal and occipital lobes when viewing the cerebral hemisphere from a medial perspective
Preoccipital sulcus	A shallow notch in the inferior surface of the cortex (superior to the cerebellum) as seen in lateral view	A surface landmark for defining the border between the parietal and occipital lobes

Contd...

Contd...

Brainstem	Comprised of: midbrain, pons and medulla oblongata	Origin of most of the cranial nerves
Midbrain	Mesencephalon	Connects forebrain and hindbrain; the site of origin of cranial nerves III and IV; contains cerebral aqueduct
Pons	Anterior portion of the metencephalon	The site of origin of cranial nerves V, VI, VII and VIII; forms part of the anterior wall of the fourth ventricle
Medulla oblongata	Also known as: myelencephalon; most caudal portion of the brainstem	It is continuous with the spinal cord at the foramen magnum; upper portion forms the floor of the fourth ventricle; the site of origin for cranial nerves VIII, IX, X, XI (cranial root), and XII

FEATURES OF THE BRAIN—INFERIOR VIEW

Structure	Description	Significance
Cerebral hemispheres	Telencephalon	Comprised of: cortex featuring gyri, sulci, fissures and lobes; commissures connecting parts; basal ganglia; contains lateral ventricles; termination of the olfactory tract (cranial nerve I)

Contd...

Contd...

Longitudinal fissure	Midline, sagittal cleft separating the paired cerebral hemispheres	Longitudinal sulcus
Frontal pole	The most anterior part of the cerebral hemisphere	Frontal pole is part of the frontal lobe
Temporal pole	The most anterior part of the temporal lobe	
Occipital pole	The most posterior part of the cerebral hemisphere	Occipital pole is part of the occipital lobe; composed of primary visual cortex
Frontal pole	Rostral to central sulcus	Contains prefrontal (emotions, personality) and precentral (primary motor) areas
Temporal lobe	Separated from the frontal lobe by the lateral sulcus	Primarily concerned with hearing and memory/learning
Occipital lobe	Posterior to an imaginary line through parieto-occipital sulcus	Contains the primarily visual cortex
Limbic lobe	Structures on the medial surface of the cerebral hemisphere which surround the rostral brainstem; includes the subcallosal gyrus, cingulate gyrus and parahippo-campal gyrus	Primarily concerned with emotions and memory
Parahippocam-pal, gyrus	Gyrus on the inferior surface of the temporal lobe that lies lateral to the midbrain	The uncus is a medial projection of the parahippocampal gyrus

Contd...

Contd...

Straight gyrus	Gyrus located on the medial side of the olfactory tract	Gyrus rectus
Lingual gyrus	Gyrus lying inferior to the calcarine sulcus	Contains primary visual cortex
Uncus	Portion of the cerebral cortex on the medial side of the parahippocampal gyrus and overlying the amygdala; located near the free edge of the tentorium cerebelli	Contains olfactory cortex
Apex of cuneus	Portion of the cuneus seen in an inferior view of the cerebral hemisphere	Contains part of the visual cortex
Longitudinal sulcus	Midline, sagittal cleft separating the paired cerebral hemispheres	Longitudinal fissure
Olfactory sulcus	Sulcus that defines the lateral margin of the straight gyrus	Contains the olfactory bulb and tract
Mamillary body	Part of the hypothalamus; a small spherical projection on the inferior surface of the floor of the third ventricle posterior to the hypophysis	Involved with memory and learning
Brainstem	Comprised of: midbrain, pons and medulla oblongata	Origin of most of the cranial nerves

Contd...

Contd...

Midbrain	Mesencephalon	Connects forebrain and hindbrain; the site of origin of cranial nerves III and IV; contains cerebral aqueduct
Pons	Anterior portion of the metencephalon	The site of origin of cranial nerves V, VI, VII and VIII; forms part of the anterior wall of the fourth ventricle
Medulla oblongata	Myelencephalon; most caudal portion of the brainstem	It is continuous with the spinal cord at the foramen magnum; upper portion forms the floor of the fourth ventricle; the site of origin for cranial nerves VIII, IX, X, XI (cranial root), and XII
Olfactory bulb	Flattened, oval enlargement at the anterior tip of the olfactory tract	Contains the olfactory mitral cells which are the origin of the axons that course through the olfactory tract; the olfactory nerve begins at the bipolar olfactory cells in the nasal mucosa and courses through the cribriform plate to the olfactory bulb
Olfactory tract	Ribbon-like nerve tract that courses from the olfactory bulb to the cerebral cortex; it courses in the olfactory sulcus	Carries the sense of smell

Contd...

Contd...

Optic chiasm	Crossover point for the nasal fibers of both retinas	Lateral visual fields (medial retinal fibers) project to the contralateral occipital lobe
Hypophysis	Midline projection of neural and endocrine tissue attached to the floor of the diencephalon	Also known as: pituitary gland

FEATURES OF THE BRAIN—MID-SAGITTAL VIEW

Structure	Description	Significance
Cerebral hemispheres	Telencephalon	Comprised of: cortex featuring gyri, sulci, fissures and lobes; commissures connecting parts; basal ganglia; contains lateral ventricles; termination of the olfactory tract (cranial nerve I)
Longitudinal fissure	Midline, sagittal cleft separating the paired cerebral hemispheres	Longitudinal sulcus; contains the falx cerebri
Frontal lobe	Rostral to central sulcus	Contains prefrontal (emotions, personality) and precentral (primary motor) areas
Parietal lobe	Separated from the frontal lobe by the central sulcus, separated from occipital lobe by line through parieto-occipital sulcus	Contains the primary and secondary somatosensory areas

Contd...

Contd...

Occipital lobe	Posterior to line through parieto-occipital sulcus	Contains the primary and secondary visual cortex
Limbic lobe	A border (limbus = Latin for border) of cortical tissue surrounding the third ventricle; comprised of: cingulate gyrus, parahippo-campal gyrus, uncus and other small portions of the adjacent cortex	Part of the brain responsible for behavior and emotions
Cingulate gyrus	The portion of the limbic lobe that lies superior to the corpus callosum	Cingulate gyrus is bounded by the callosal sulcus and the cingulate sulcus
Straight gyrus	Gyrus located on the medial side of the olfactory tract	Gyrus rectus
Lingual gyrus	The portion of the occipital lobe that lies inferior to the calcarine sulcus	Cortical projection of the upper half of the contralateral visual field
Cingulate sulcus	The sulcus that lies superior to the cingulate gyrus	
Central sulcus	Separates the frontal lobe from the parietal lobe; separates sensory cortex from motor cortex	Fissure of Rolando
Parieto-occipital sulcus	Sulcus on the medial surface of the cerebral hemisphere that lies between the precuneus and the cuneus	Forms the boundary between the parietal lobe and the occipital lobe

Contd...

Contd...

Calcarine sulcus	Sulcus between the lingual gyrus and the cuneus	Primary visual cortex is both superior and inferior to it
Cuneus	Part of the cerebral cortex that forms the upper wall of the calcarine fissure	Cortical projection of the lower half of the contralateral visual field
Pineal gland	Pineal body	Represents an endocrine gland attached to diencephalon
Corpus callosum	Midline part of great cerebral commissure	Connects paired cerebral hemispheres
Anterior commissure	A bundle of association fibers located anterior to the third ventricle	Connections between the left and right temporal lobes
Posterior commissure	A bundle of association fibers located posterior to the third ventricle, just inferior to the pineal gland	Connections between various areas of the right and left sides of the midbrain
Optic chiasm	Crossover point for the nasal fibers of both retinas	Lateral visual fields (medial retinal fibers) project to the contralateral occipital lobe
Thalamus	An egg-shaped collection of nuclei forming part of the lateral wall of the third ventricle	Distributes information to appropriate areas of the cerebral cortex
Hypothalamus	A collection on nuclei forming the anterior portion of the lateral wall of the third ventricle	Controls visceral activity and elicits phenomena associated with the emotions
Body of fornix	A group of nerve cell fibers arching beneath the corpus callosum	Main efferent fiber system of the hippocampal formation

Contd...

Contd...

Hypophysis	Midline projection of neural and endocrine tissue attached to the floor of the diencephalon	Pituitary gland
Brainstem	Comprised of: midbrain, pons and medulla oblongata	Origin of most of the cranial nerves
Midbrain	Mesencephalon	Connects forebrain and hindbrain; the site of origin of cranial nerves III and IV; contains cerebral aqueduct
Pons	Anterior portion of the metencephalon	The site of origin of cranial nerves V, VI, VII and VIII; forms part of the anterior wall of the fourth ventricle
Medulla oblongata	Myelencephalon; most caudal portion of the brainstem	It is continuous with the spinal cord at the foramen magnum; upper portion forms the floor of the fourth ventricle; the site of origin for cranial nerves VIII, IX, X, XI (cranial root), and XII
Cerebellum	Posterior part of metencephalon	Largest part of hindbrain; important for coordination of movement

FEATURES OF THE BRAINSTEM

Structure	Description	Significance
Midbrain	Mesencephalon	Connects forebrain and hindbrain; site of origin of cranial nerves III and IV; contains cerebral aqueduct

Contd...

Contd...

Pons	Anterior portion of metencephalon	Site of origin of cranial nerves V, VI, VII and VIII; forms part of the anterior wall of the fourth ventricle
Medulla oblongata	Myelencephalon; most caudal portion of brainstem	Continuous with the spinal cord at the foramen magnum; upper portion forms the floor of the fourth ventricle; site of origin for cranial nerves IX, X, XI (cranial root), and XII

SURFACE FEATURES OF THE BRAINSTEM AS SEEN ON MID-SAGITTAL VIEW

Structure	Description	Significance
Midbrain		
Tectum	The roof of the midbrain, formed by the superior and inferior colliculi; located dorsal to the cerebral aqueduct	Also known as: quadrigeminal plate
Superior colliculus	Paired elevations of midbrain tectum	Part of corpora quadrigemina; important for reflex movements of eye, head and neck
Inferior colliculus	Paired elevations of midbrain tectum	Part of corpora quadrigemina; important for auditory reflexes
Tegmentum	The collection of cells and nerve fibers located ventral to the ventricle	Gives rise to the middle cerebellar peduncle

Contd...

Contd...

	system in the midbrain, pons and medulla	
Cerebral aqueduct	Canal connecting third and fourth ventricles, passing through midbrain	Also known as: aqueduct of Sylvius
Pons		
Fourth ventricle	Midline space between cerebellum posteriorly and pons and upper medulla anteriorly	Communicates anterosuperiorly with third ventricle via cerebral aqueduct; drains CSF via median aperature and lateral aperatures
Central canal of spinal cord	Small opening in the center of the spinal cord	Continuous with the central canal of the medulla and, through it, with the fourth ventricle of the brain

VENTRICULAR SYSTEM OF THE BRAIN

Structure	*Description*	*Significance*
Lateral ventricle	Paired spaces within cerebral hemispheres	They drain cerebrospinal fluid to the third ventricle via the interventricular foramina (of Monro)
Third ventricle	Midline space within the diencephalon between the paired dorsal thalami and the hypothalamus	Communicates rostrolaterally with paired lateral ventricles via interventricular foramina, communicates posteroinferiorly with fourth ventricle via cerebral aqueduct

Contd...

Contd...

Fourth ventricle	Midline space between cerebellum posteriorly and pons and upper medulla anteriorly	Communicates anterosuperiorly with third ventricle via cerebral aqueduct; drains CSF via median aperature and lateral aperatures
Choroid plexus	Vascular membranes that occur within the ventricles	Production of cerebrospinal fluid
Interventricular foramen	Communication between the lateral ventricle and the third ventricle; paired, one on each side	Also known as: foramina of Monro
Cerebral aqueduct	Canal connecting third and fourth ventricles, passing through midbrain	Also known as: aqueduct of Sylvius
Median aperature	Midline, irregular foramen draining fourth ventricle posteroinferiorly into cerebellomedullary cistern	Also known as: foramen of Magendie
Lateral aperature	Paired foramina draining fourth ventricle laterally into cerebellomedullary cistern	Also known as: foramina of Luschka
Central canal of spinal cord	Small opening in the center of the spinal cord	Continuous with the central canal of the medulla and, through it, with the fourth ventricle of the brain

BLOOD SUPPLY TO THE BRAIN

Artery	Source	Branches	Supply to	Notes
Anterior spinal	Contributions received from several arteries (vertebral, posterior intercostal, subcostal, lumbar, lateral sacral aa.)	Pial arterial plexus	Meninges; spinal cord; medulla (dorsal motor nucleus of cranial nerve X, nucleus ambiguous, spinal accessory nucleus and hypoglossal nucleus)	Anterior spinal artery anastomoses with the nterior radicular brs. of the spinal rami of the vertebral, posterior intercostal, subcostal, lumbar and lateral sacral artery
Basilar	Formed by the joining of the two vertebral aa.	Pontine brs., anterior inferior cerebellar a., superior cerebellar a., two posterior cerebral aa. (terminal brs.)	Pons (motor nucleus of cranial nerve V, chief sensory nucleus of cranial nerve V, abducens nucleus, facial nucleus, superior salivatory nucleus); oculomotor nucleus; nucleus of Edinger-Westphal; cerebellum; posterior cerebrum	Basilar a. contributes blood to the cerebral arterial circle
Cerebellar, anterior inferior	Basilar a.	Labyrinthine a. (usually)	Pons (motor nucleus of cranial nerve V, chief sensory nucleus of cranial nerve V, abducens nucleus, facial nucleus, superior salivatory nucleus); cerebellum; inner ear	Anterior inferior cerebella a. shares its region of supply with branches of the basilar a.

Contd...

Contd...

Cerebellar, posterior inferior	Vertebral a.	Posterior spinal a.	Part of cerebellum; medulla (cochlear nucleus, vestibular nucleus, dorsal motor nucleus of cranial nerve X, nucleus ambiguous)	Posterior inferior cerebellar a. shares its region of supply with the vertebral a. and anterior spinal a. (watershed region)
Cerebellar, superior	Basilar a.	No named branches	Upper cerebellum; trochlear nucleus	There may be more than one superior cerebellar a. arising from the basilar a. on each side
Cerebral, anterior	Internal carotid a.	Anterior communicating a., medial frontobasal a., polar frontal a., callosomarginal a., precuneal a.	Medial and inferior portions of the frontal lobe; medial side of the parietal lobe; corpus callosum and part of the limbic lobe; olfactory bulb and tract; optic nerve, optic chiasm and optic tract	The anterior communicating a. unites the two anterior cerebral aa. across the midline
Cerebral arterial circle	An anastomotic circle of blood vessels formed by portions of the following vessels: posterior cerebral aa. (2); posterior communicating aa. (2); internal carotid aa. (2); anterior cerebral aa. (2); anterior communicating a.	This is an anastomotic loop; major named vessels connect here, but there are no named branches of the arterial circle	Brain and midbrain	Also known as: arterial circle of Willis

Contd...

Contd...

Middle cerebral	Internal carotid a.	Lateral frontobasal a.; prefrontal sulcal a.; precentral sulcal a.; central sulcal a.; anterior parietal a.; posterior parietal a.; anterior, middle and posterior temporal aa.	Frontal, parietal and temporal lobes, especially on their lateral surfaces	The middle cerebral a. is the direct continuation of the internal carotid a.
Posterior cerebral	Basilar a.	Posterior cerebral a.; anterior and posterior temporal brs.; medial occipital a.	Part of the brainstem (oculomotor nucleus, nucleus of Edinger-Westphal, trochlear nucleus); medial and inferior portions of the temporal lobe; occipital lobe	The two posterior cerebral aa. are the terminal brs. of the basilar a.
Anterior communicating	Anterior cerebral a.	Perforating aa.	An anastomotic connection	Anterior communicating a. is a short vessel of anastomosis which crosses the midline to join the paired anterior cerebral aa.; it is part of the Circle of Willis
Posterior communicating	Internal carotid a.	Perforating aa.	An anastomotic connection	A vessel of anastomosis which connects the internal carotid a. to the posterior cerebral a.; part of the cerebral arterial circle (of Willis)

Contd...

Contd...

Ophthalmic	Internal carotid a.	Central retinal a., lacrimal a., muscular brs., anterior ethmoidal a., posterior ethmoidal a., medial palpebral a., supraorbital a., supratrochlear a., dorsal nasal a.	Optic nerve, optic chiasm optic tract, retina, extraocular mm., eyelids, forehead, ethmoidal air cells, lateral nasal wall, dorsum of the nose	Ophthalmic a. provides the only artery to the retina (central retinal a.)
Vertebral	Subclavian a. (1st part)	Spinal brs., muscular brs., anterior spinal a., posterior inferior cerebellar a., medullary brs., meningeal brs., basilar a.	Deep neck, cervical spinal cord, spinal cord; medulla (dorsal motor nucleus of cranial nerve X, nucleus ambiguus, spinal accessory nucleus and hypoglossal nucleus)	Vertebral a. anastomoses with the internal carotid a. in the cerebral arterial circle (of Willis); it courses through the transverse foramina of vertebrae C1-C6
Anterior spinal	Contributions received from several arteries (vertebral, posterior intercostal, subcostal, lumbar, lateral sacral aa.)	Pial arterial plexus	Meninges; spinal cord; medulla (dorsal motor nucleus of cranial nerve X, nucleus ambiguous, spinal accessory nucleus and hypoglossal nucleus)	The anterior spinal a. anastomoses with the anterior radicular brs. of the spinal rami of the vertebral, posterior intercostal, subcostal, lumbar and lateral sacral aa.

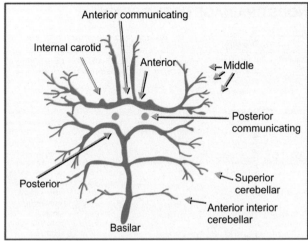

FIGURE 1.1: Diagram showing the circle of Willis

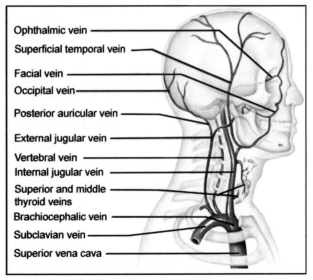

FIGURE 1.2: Schematic for neck veins

VENOUS DRAINAGE OF THE BRAIN

Vein	Tributaries	Drains into	Regions Drained	Notes
Great cerebral	Formed by the union of the paired internal cerebral vv.	Straight sinus	Deep portions of the cerebrum	Great cerebral v. is a very short vessel
Inferior cerebral	Tributaries are unnamed	Cavernous sinus, transverse sinus, superior petrosal sinus	Inferior aspect of the cerebral hemispheres	Inferior cerebral vv. are numerous
Superiorc cerebral	Tributaries are unnamed	Superior sagittal sinus	Superior aspect of the cerebral hemispheres	Superior cerebral vv. bleed into the subdural space when injured, resulting in a subdural hematoma; also known as: bridging vv.
Inferior sagittal sinus	Unnamed tributaries from the falx cerebri and cerebral hemispheres	Unites with the great cerebral v. to form the straight sinus	Medial surfaces fo the cerebral hemispheres	Inferior sagittal sinus is directly superior to the corpus callosum in the free margin of falx cerebri
Inferior petrosal sinus	Cavernous sinus	Sigmoid sinus, at its distal end	All regions drained by the cavernous sinus, including the orbit and brain	Inferior petrosal sinus lies within the dura mater along the inferior portion of the petrous part of the temporal bone
Occipital sinus	No named tributaries	Confluens of sinuses	Cerebellum	Lies within the dura mater at the base of the falx cerebelli

Contd...

Contd...

Superior petrosal sinus	Cavernous sinus	Sigmoid sinus, at its proximal end	All regions drained by the cavernous sinus, including the orbit and brain	Superior petrosal sinus lies on the petrous ridge within the dura mater at the line of attachment of the tentorium cerebelli
Superior sagittal sinus	V. of the foramen cecum; superior cerebral vv.	Confluens of sinuses	Cerebral hemispheres	Superior sagittal sinus occupies the superior part of the falx cerebri; lateral lacunae receive grossly visible arachnoid granulations
Straight sinus	Inferior sagittal sinus, great cerebral vein, superior cerebellar vv.	Confluens of sinuses	deep parts of the cerebrum, cerebellum	Straight sinus lies within the junction of the falx cerebri and tentorium cerebelli; also known as: sinus rectus
Transverse sinus	Confluence of sinuses, inferior cerebral vv.	Sigmoid sinus	Brain	Lies within the line of attachment of the tentorium cerebelli to the inner surface of the calvaria

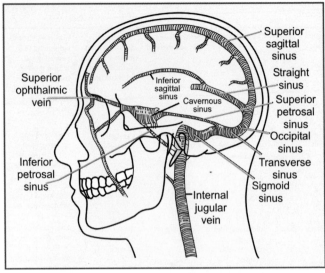

FIGURE 1.3: Schematic showing dural venous sinuses

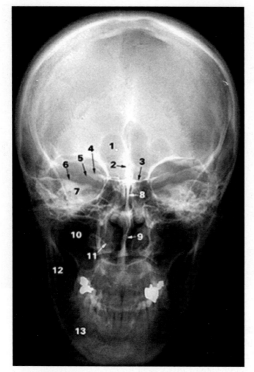

FIGURE 1.4: Frontal radiograph of skull

1. Frontal sinus
2. Crista galli
3. Cribriform plate
4. Lesser wing of sphenoid
5. Superior orbital fissure
6. Superior border of petrous part of temporal bone
7. Dense shadow of petrous part of temporal bone
8. Perpendicular plate of the ethmoid
9. Vomer
10. Maxillary sinus
11. Inferior concha
12. Ramus of mandible
13. Body of mandible

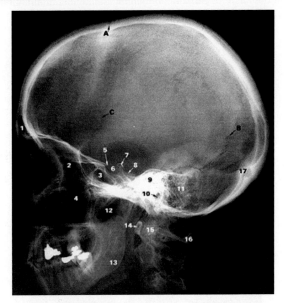

FIGURE 1.5: Lateral radiograph of skull

1. Frontal sinus
2. Ethmoidal sinus
3. Sphenoidal sinus
4. Maxillary sinus
5. Anterior clinoid processes
6. Hypophyseal fossa
7. Posterior clinoid processes
8. Clivus
9. Great density of the petrous part of the temporal bone
10. External acoustic meatus
11. Mastoid cells
12. Nasopharynx
13. Angle of mandible
14. Anterior arch of the atlas
15. Dens of axis
16. Posterior arch of the atlas
17. Internal occipital protuberance
    A. Coronal suture
    B. Lambdoid suture
    C. The grooves for the branches of the middle meningeal vessels

AXIAL ANATOMY—BRAIN

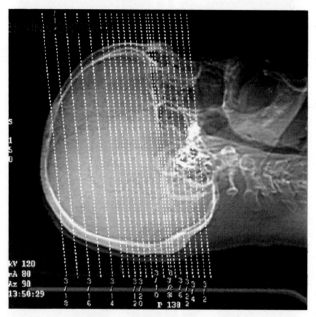

FIGURE 1.6: Digital scanogram brain

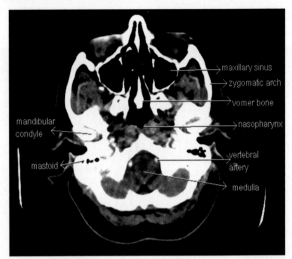

FIGURE 1.7: Axial CT at the level of medulla

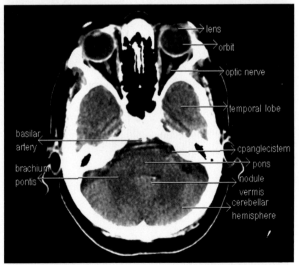

FIGURE 1.8: Axial CT at the level of pons

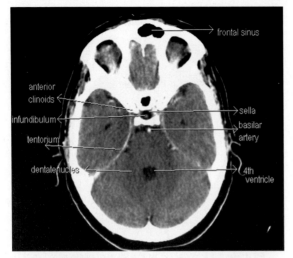

FIGURE 1.9: Axial CT at the level of sella

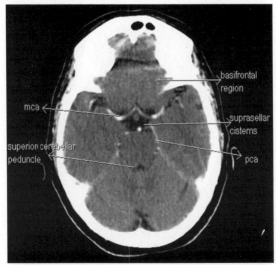

FIGURE 1.10: Axial CT at the level of suprasellar cistern

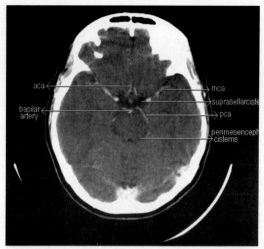

FIGURE 1.11: Axial CT at the level of circle of Willis

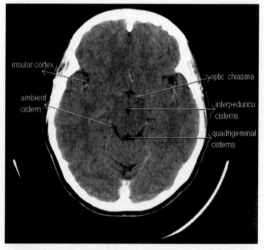

FIGURE 1.12: Axial CT at the level of tentorial hiatus

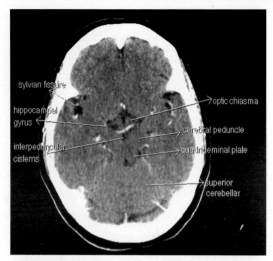

FIGURE 1.13: Axial CT at the level of optic chiasma

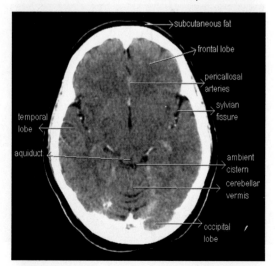

FIGURE 1.14: Axial CT at the level of ambient cistern

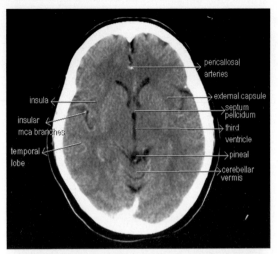

FIGURE 1.15: Axial CT at the level of third ventricle

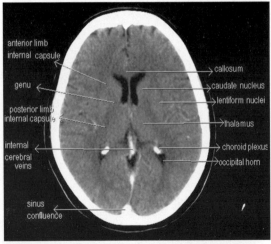

FIGURE 1.16: Axial Ct at the level of basal ganglia

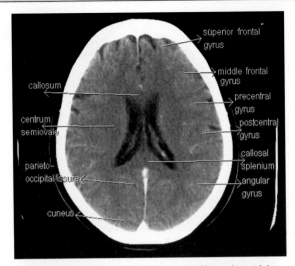

FIGURE 1.17: Axial CT at the level of lateral ventricle

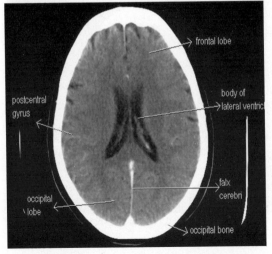

FIGURE 1.18: Axial CT at the level of corona

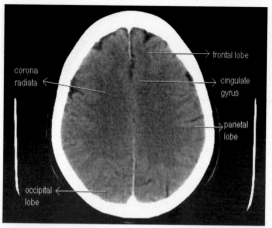

FIGURE 1.19: Axial CT at the supraventricular level

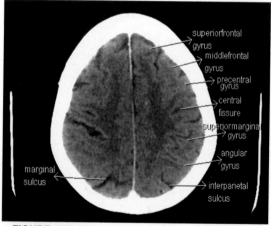

FIGURE 1.20: Axial CT at the level of central fissure

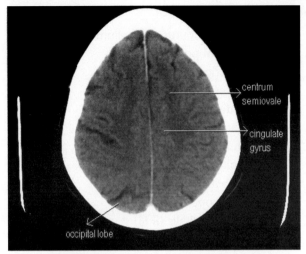

FIGURE 1.21: Axial CT at the level of centrum

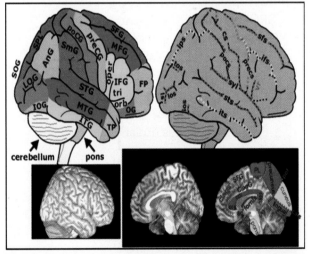

FIGURE 1.22: Schematic diagram showing the various sulci and gyri

NAMED GYRI AND SULCI

AnG	angular gyrus cerebellum
FP	frontal pole
IFG	inferior frontal gyrus
IOG	inferior occipital gyrus
ITG	inferior temporal gyrus
LOG	lateral occipital gyrus
MFG	middle frontal gyrus
MTG	middle temporal gyrus
OG	orbital gyrus pons
oper	pars opercularis (IFG)
orb	pars orbitalis (IFG)
tri	pars triangularis (IFG)
poCG	postcentral gyrus
preCG	precentral gyrus
SFG	superior frontal gyrus
SOG	superior occipital gyrus
SPL	superior parietal lobe
STG	superior temporal gyrus
SmG	supramarginal gyrus
TP	temporal pole
cs	central sulcus (Rolandic)
hr	horizontal ramus
ifs	inferior frontal sulcus
ios	inferior occipital sulcus
ips	intraparietal sulcus
syl	lateral fissure (Sylvian)
los	lateral occipital sulcus
ls	lunate sulcus

pof	parieto-occipital fissure
pocs	postcentral sulcus
precs	precentral sulcus
sfs	superior frontal sulcus
tos	transoccipital sulcus
vr	vertical ramus
ac	anterior commissure
cals	calcarine sulcus
cings	cingulate sulcus
CingG	cingulate gyrus
ccb	corpus callosum (body)
ccg	corpus callosum (genu)
ccs	corpus callosum (splenium)
	cuneus
	fornix
lingual	lingual gyrus
mb	mamillary bodies
PL	paracentral lobule precuneus
q	quadrigeminal plate

Chapter 2

Temporal Bone

The temporal bone contains the sensory organs of hearing and balance, and structurally contributes to the cranial vault. The temporal bone consists of five parts: the squamous, the mastoid, the tympanic, zygomatic and petrous segment. It contains portions of the carotid artery and jugular venous drainage system, and is intimately related to the dura of the middle and posterior fossa. Anteriorly, it articulates with the condyle of the mandible. Posteriorly, and superiorly, the mastoid air cell system communicates with the middle ear. The facial nerve passes through the temporal bone en route to the muscles of facial expression.

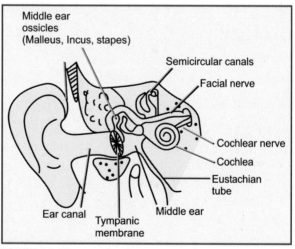

FIGURE 2.1: Diagram showing structure of auditory apparatus

THE EAR

Both functionally and anatomically, the ear can be divided into three parts.

EXTERNAL EAR

That portion external to the tympanic membrane. It serves chiefly to protect the tympanic membrane, but also collects and directs sound waves and plays a role in sound localization. The skin of the external ear normally migrates laterally from the umbo of the malleus in the tympanic membrane to the external auditory meatus (at a rate of 2-3 mm per day). This is a unique and essential mechanism for maintaining patency of the canal.

The Auricle

Elastic cartilage covered with closely adherent skin. The configuration is intricate, and extremely difficult to duplicate.

External Auditory Canal

- **Lateral portion**—Cartilaginous with thick, loosely applied skin containing ceruminous and sebaceous glands.
- **Medial portion**—Very thin skin directly over bone, no skin appendages. Curves anteriorly and medially in adults, which may obscure the anterior tympanic membrane. It comprises two-thirds of the total canal in adults, less in infants and children.

THE MIDDLE EAR

This is an air-containing space which communicates with the nasopharynx via the eustachian tube. It is normally sealed laterally by the tympanic membrane. Its function is

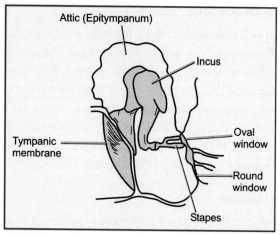

FIGURE 2.2: Schematic diagram of middle ear structures

to transmit and amplify sound waves from tympanic membrane to the stapes footplate converting energy from air medium to a fluid medium of the membranous labyrinth. The relationship of the three ossicles is depicted below.

LEFT EAR VIEWED POSTERIORLY

- **The tympanic membrane** is an ovoid, three-layered structure consisting of squamous epithelium laterally, respiratory mucosa medially, and an intervening fibrous layer. It normally has a conical shape, with the apex maintained medially by the support of the malleus. The fibrous layer thickens laterally to form the annulus, an incomplete ring which is attached to surrounding bone. Superior to the lateral process of the malleus,

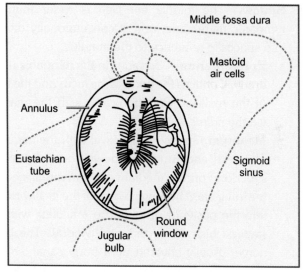

FIGURE 2.3: Schematic diagram of tympanic membrane

this ring is deficient, and this area is known as the pars flaccida. The majority of the drum is composed of the pars tensa.

- **Ossicles**—Three small bones which are involved in sound conduction. From lateral to medial, these are the malleus, the incus, and the stapes. The handle and lateral process of the malleus is attached to the tympanic membrane and can be easily seen on physical exam. The long process of the incus can often be seen through the posterior superior quadrant of the membrane. The stapes is attached to a footplate which is in direct contact with the fluid of the inner ear (See Figures 2.1 and 2.3).

- **Spaces**—The middle ear cleft is wider than the tympanic membrane, and is conventionally divided into spaces in reference to the annulus.
  - **Epitympanum**—Superior to the tympanic membrane. Contains the body of the incus and the head of the malleus. Communicates with the mastoid via the *aditus*.
  - **Mesotympanum**—On a level with the eardrum. The oval and round windows, located postero-superiorly on the medial wall, communicate with the inner ear. The long process of the incus projects into the posterior quadrant to articulate with the stapes which sits in the oval window. The facial nerve, usually covered by a bony canal, crosses the posterior superior quadrant superior to the stapes, then courses inferiorly between the middle ear and mastoid air cells.
  - **Protympanum**—In this anterior recess of the middle ear, the eustachian tube exits to communicate with the nasopharynx. This tube runs in close proximity to the carotid artery.
  - **Hypotympanum**—The jugular bulb curves through the hypotympanum. It is usually covered by bone, but may be dehiscent and extend into the middle ear space.

INNER EAR

Consists of a fluid-filled labyrinth which functions to convert mechanical energy into neural impulses. The *bony*

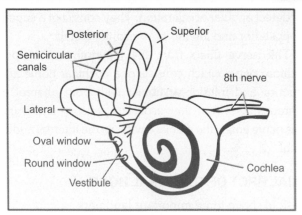

FIGURE 2.4: Diagram of vestibulo-cochlear apparatus

labyrinth is subdivided into smaller compartments by the *membranous* labyrinth. Fluid surrounding the membranous labyrinth is called perilymph; fluid within is called endolymph. There are three main divisions of the bony labyrinth.

- **Vestibule**—Just medial to the oval window, and contains the utricle and the saccule, two organs of balance. The vestibule is an antechamber, leading to both the cochlear and the semicircular canal.
- **The cochlea**—A snail-shaped chamber anterior to the vestibule. It bulges into the middle ear and its bony covering is the *promontory*. The cochlea also communicates with the middle ear via the round window. In this organ, sound waves are converted into neural impulses with elaborate coding.
- **The Semicircular canals**—Three in number; project posteriorly from the vestibule. These organs

detect angular acceleration. They consist of a superior, posterior and lateral, or horizontal canals.

The nerve fibers from the labyrinth make up the auditory nerve which consists of a cochlear nerve and a superior and inferior vestibular with both afferent and efferent fibers from the respective sensory end organs. This nerve enters the cranial cavity via the internal auditory canal.

AXIAL HRCT OF TEMPORAL BONE

Mastoid have three important landmark

1. The antrum
2. Aditus and antrum
3. Koerners septum.

The aditus connects the epitympanum (attic) to the mastoid antrum. Koerners septum is part of the petro-squamous suture that runs posterolaterally through the mastoid air cells.

Middle ear cavity—is divided to epitympanum (attic), mesotympanum (tympanic cavity proper) hypotym-panum. The roof of middle ear cavity is the tegmen tympani, the tympanic membrane forms the lateral wall of the middle-ear cavity. Inferiorly the middle ear is in relation to the jugular bulb. The medial wall is the labyrinthine wall were the oval window, round window and the cochlear promontory is situated the anterior wall is in relation to the carotid canal the posterior wall is formed by the mastoid.

Epitympanum on coronal section is that portion of the middle ear cavity above the line drawn between the inferior tip of scutum and the tympanic portion of the facal nerve canal. This is the site for the malleus and incus giving rise to the icecone sign.

Prussaks space— area between the incus and the lateral side wall of the epitympanum within the mesotympanum lies the rest of the ossicles.

Inner ear—the bony labyrinth houses the cochlea, vestibule semicircular canals, the vestibular and cochlear aqueducts. The cochlea is situated anteroinferiorly to the vestibule and resembles a snail shell with two and three quarter turns the cochlear aqueduct runs medial to lateral from the basal turn of the cochlea to the lateral border of the jugular foramen.

Vestibule is seen as a rounded lucency in the bony labyrinth situated lateral and posterior to the fundus of the aim the semicircular canal projects from the superior, posterior and lateral aspect of the vestibule the superior semicircular canal projects on the petrous pyramid producing the arcuate eminence. The vestibular aqueduct is seen coursing posteroinferiorly to the posterior wall of the petrous pyramid as hockey stick lucency.

TEMPORAL BONE – AXIAL HIGH RESOLUTION SECTIONS

See Figures 2.5 to 2.16.

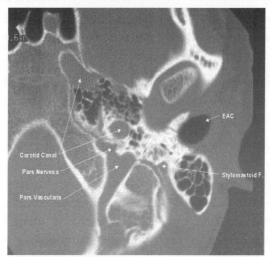

FIGURE 2.5: Axial CT at the level of stylomastoid foramina

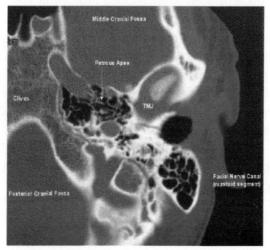

FIGURE 2.6: Axial CT at the level of fascial nerve canal

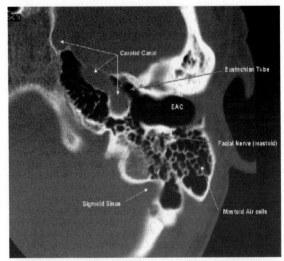

FIGURE 2.7: Axial CT at the level of external auditory canal

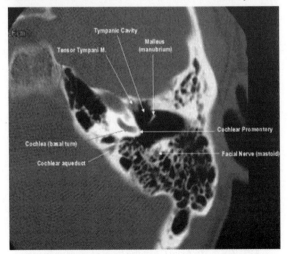

FIGURE 2.8: Axial CT at the level of tympanic cavity

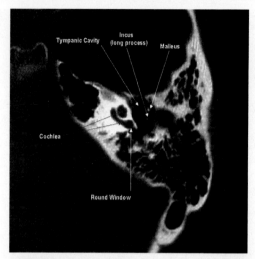

FIGURE 2.9: Axial CT at the level of round window

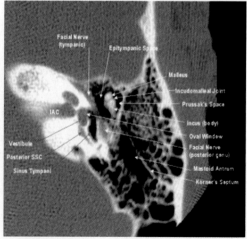

FIGURE 2.10: Axial CT at the level of malleus/incus

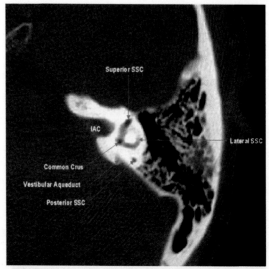

FIGURE 2.11: Axial CT at the level of semicircular canals

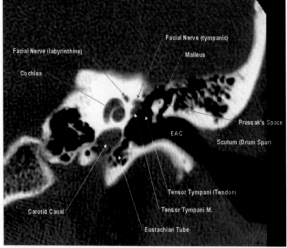

FIGURE 2.12: Coronal CT at the level of external auditory canal

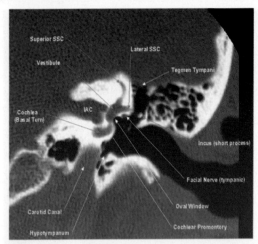

FIGURE 2.13: Coronal CT at the level of internal auditory meatus

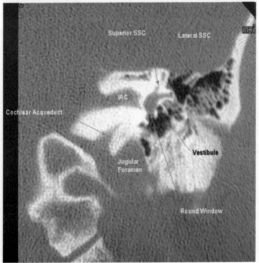

FIGURE 2.14: Coronal CT at the level of jugular foramen

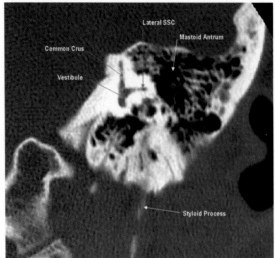

FIGURE 2.15: Coronal CT at the level of styloid process

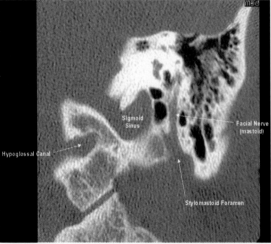

FIGURE 2.16: Coronal CT at the level of stylomastoid foramen

Chapter 3

Paranasal Sinuses

The paransal sinuses are air containing spaces within the facial bones which in part form the floor of the anterior cranial fossa and skull base. These air containing spaces are located in the frontal bones (frontal sinuses), maxillary bone (maxillary sinuses) sphenoid bone (sphenoid sinuses) ethmoid bones (ethmoid sinuses). These air sinuses communicate with each other and with the nasal passages through openings under the superior and middle turbinates.

The radiological evaluation of nasal cavity and the paranasal sinuses should stress the display of osteomeatal units (omu) omu comprises of the maxillary sinus ostium,

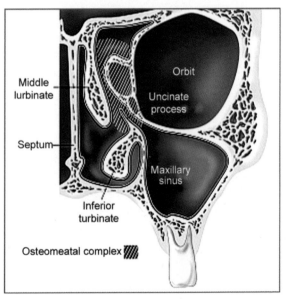

FIGURE 3.1

the ethmoid infundibulum, anterior ethmoid cells, and the frontal recess. These aerated channels provide airflow to and mucociliary clearance from the frontal, maxillary, anterior, middle ethmoidal and sphenoid sinuses.

The lateral nasal walls contains three bulbous projections—the superior, middle, and inferior turbinate. The turbinates serve to divide the passages into superior, middle and inferior meatus.

Superior meatus—drains the posterior ethmoid cells, and the sphenoid sinus (via the sphenoethmoidal recess) the middle meatus receives drainage from the frontal sinus (via frontal recess) maxillary sinus (via the maxillary ostium and ethmoid infundibulum) and the anterior ethmoid aircells (via ethmoid ostia and frontal recess) the inferior meatus receives drainage from the nasolacrimal duct.

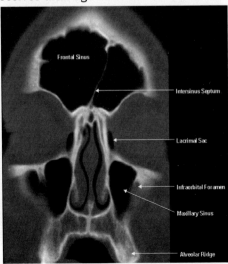

FIGURE 3.2: Coronal CT at the level of frontal sinus

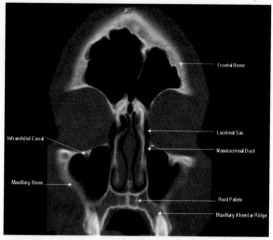

FIGURE 3.3: Coronal CT at the level of nasolacrimal duct

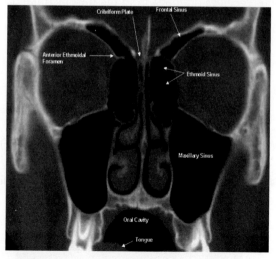

FIGURE 3.4: Coronal CT at the level of maxillary sinus

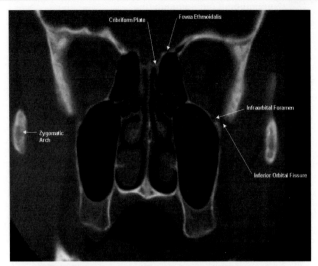

FIGURE 3.5: Coronal CT at the level of cribriform plate

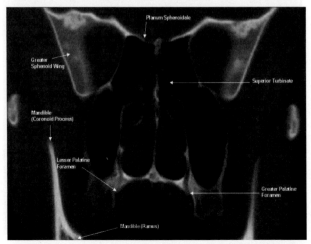

FIGURE 3.6: Coronal CT at the level of planum sphenoidale

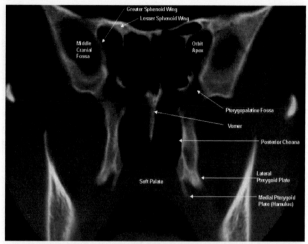

FIGURE 3.7: Coronal CT at the level of obital apex

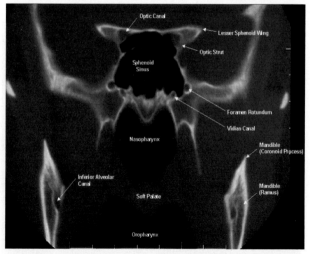

FIGURE 3.8: Coronal CT at the level of sphenoid sinus

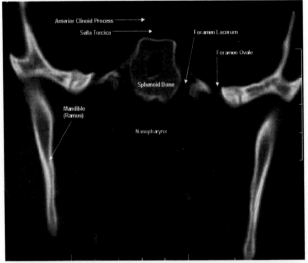

FIGURE 3.9: Coronal CT at the level of foramen ovale

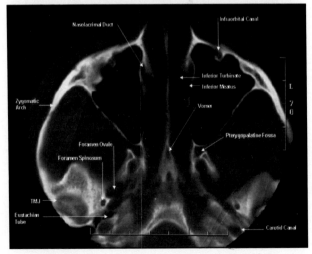

FIGURE 3.10: Axial CT at the level of maxillary sinus

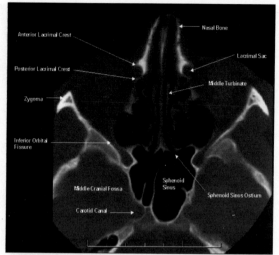

FIGURE 3.11: Axial CT at the level of sphenoid sinus

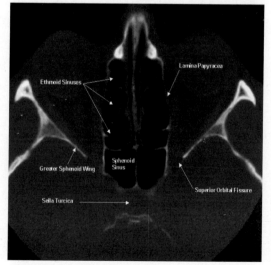

FIGURE 3.12: Axial CT at the level of ethmoid sinus

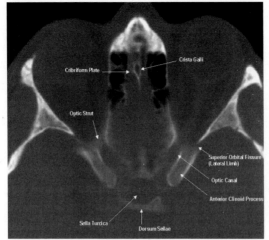

FIGURE 3.13: Axial CT at the level of cribriform plate

Chapter 4

Neck

The neck contains important communications between the head and the body, including air and food passages, major blood vessels and nerves, and the spinal cord. Many vital structures are compressed into a narrow area which is engineered for maximal mobility to permit variation in head position relative to body.

SKELETON

Primarily composed of the vertebral column. Anteriorly, the hyoid bone, and laryngeal and tracheal cartilages support the aerodigestive spaces. These are suspended from the mandible and base of skull by a system of muscles and ligaments.

MUSCLES

Anteriorly, strap muscles connect the respiratory skeleton and sternum. There are also muscular attachments from the hyoid to the tongue, mandible, and styloid. The digastric muscle passes forward from the mastoid, attaches to the hyoid, then ascends to the anterior mandible. The sterno-cleidomastoid (SCM) divides the neck into anterior and posterior triangles. The posterior triangle is largely muscular. The anterior triangle which contains most of the vital structures, can be divided into smaller triangles by muscles.

The anterior and posterior bellies of the digastric form the submandibular triangle. The submental triangle is in the midline, between the anterior bellies. The vascular or carotid triangle is inferior to the digastric and hyoid.

The omohyoid is a small muscle, running at roughly 90 degrees to the SCM, from the hyoid to the scapula.

NERVES

The neck contains major branches of cranial nerves, as well as cervical roots.

CRANIAL NERVES

- **VII**—The marginal mandibular branch dips down into the neck in the fascia overlying the submandibular gland. In addition to the muscles of facial expression, branches of VII innervate the platysma, the stylohyoid and the posterior belly of the digastric.
- **X**—The vagus nerve exits the jugular foramen and travels inferiorly in the carotid sheath. It carries the parasympathetic fibers of the thoracic cavity and much of the GI tract, as well as laryngeal and pharyngeal sensory and motor branches.
- **The Spinal Accessory Nerve (XI)**—Supplies the trapezius and sternocleidomastoid muscles. It exits the jugular foramen, then runs posteriorly.
- **The Hypoglossal Nerve (XII)**—Supplies the muscles of the tongue. The nerve exits the skull through its own canal, runs downward in the carotid sheath, then curves forward superficially to the carotid at the level of the occipital artery to reach the tongue.

CERVICAL NERVES

- Cervical plexus—anterior roots of C1-4
  - Ansa cervicalis—to strap muscles (some travel with XII)
  - Branches to phrenic nerve
  - Sensory
- Phrenic nerve - C3-5
- Brachial Plexus C5-T1
- Posterior rami - to posterior muscles and skin
- Cervical sympathetic chain - travels in carotid sheath

MAJOR VASCULAR STRUCTURES

- Carotid artery—bifurcates into:
  - Internal (intracranial)—no branches in the neck
  - External (extracranial)—branches:
    - Superior thyroid
    - Ascending pharyngeal
    - Lingual
    - Facial
    - Occipital
    - Post-auricular
    - Superficial temporal
    - Internal maxillary
  - Thyrocervical trunk
    - Suprascapular
    - Transverse cervical
    - Inferior thyroid
  - Vertebral artery

- Internal jugular vein (within carotid sheath)
- External jugular vein

VISCERAL COLUMN

Pharynx, larynx, trachea, and esophagus.

THYROID GLAND

- Developmentally derived from pharyngeal floor
- Located anterior and lateral to the trachea
- Closely related to recurrent laryngeal nerve and parathyroid glands
- Blood supply
  - Arterial
    - Superior thyroid artery (branch of external carotid)
    - Inferior thyroid artery (branch of thyrocervical trunk)
    - Thyroid "ima" artery (variable)
  - Venous
    - Superior thyroid vein
    - Middle thyroid vein
    - Inferior thyroid vein

PARATHYROID GLANDS

- Four glands: two on each side
- Derived from branchial pouches III and IV: Superior parathyroid glands from pouch IV and inferior parathyroid gland from pouch III.

- Glands usually related to posterior surface of thyroid gland, but may be found as inferior as mediastinum

ANATOMIC TRIANGLES (superimposed on superficial neck anatomy)

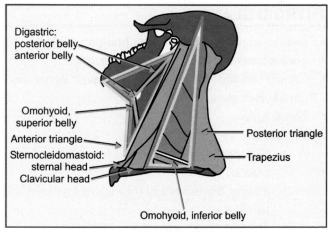

Digastric:
posterior belly
anterior belly

Omohyoid,
superior belly

Anterior triangle

Sternocleidomastoid:
sternal head
Clavicular head

Posterior triangle

Trapezius

Omohyoid, inferior belly

FIGURE 4.1: Schematics of triangles of neck

The neck can be divided into two major triangles, with multiple smaller triangles:

ANTERIOR TRIANGLE

Bordered by the anterior border of the SCM, midline of the neck, and the mandible

- **Muscular triangle**—formed by the midline, superior belly of the omohyoid, and SCM
- **Carotid triangle**—formed by the superior belly of the omohyoid, SCM, and posterior belly of the digastric

- **submental triangle**—formed by the anterior belly of the digastric, hyoid, and midline
- **submandibular triangle**—formed by the mandible, posterior belly of the digastric, and anterior belly of the digastric

POSTERIOR TRIANGLE

Bordered by the posterior border of the SCM, trapezius, and clavicle:

- **Supraclavicular triangle**—formed by the inferior belly of the omohyoid, clavicle, and SCM
- **Occipital triangle**—formed by inferior belly of the omohyoid, trapezius, and SCM

Lymphatic Drainage

Major head and neck lymph node groups.

The lymph nodes of the neck can be divided into six levels within the defined anatomic triangles. These groups and the areas that they drain are particularly important when locating and working up a "neck mass" or possible malignancy. The groups and drainage areas are as follows:

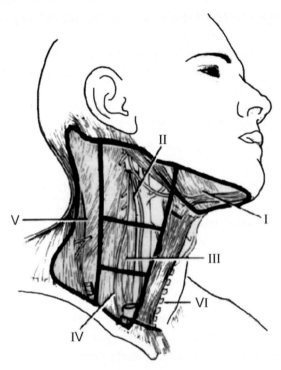

FIGURE 4.2: Diagram showing level of neck nodes

- I—Submental and submandibular nodes
- II—Upper jugulodigastric group
- III—Middle jugular nodes draining the naso- and oropharynx, oral cavity, hypopharynx, larynx.
- IV—Inferior jugular nodes draining the hypopharynx, subglottic larynx, thyroid, and esophagus.
- V— Posterior triangle group
- VI—Anterior compartment group

INDIVIDUAL LYMPH NODES IN THE HEAD AND NECK

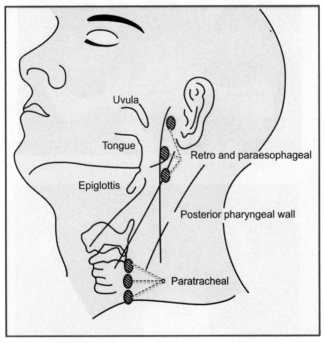

FIGURE 4.3

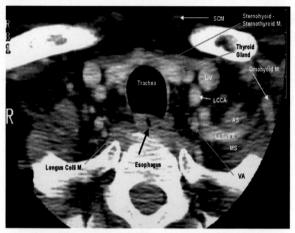

FIGURE 4.4: Axial CT section at the level of trachea

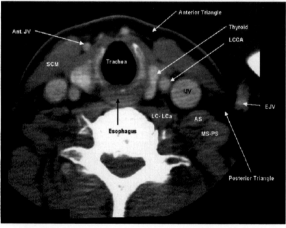

FIGURE 4.5: Axial CT section at the level of thyroid

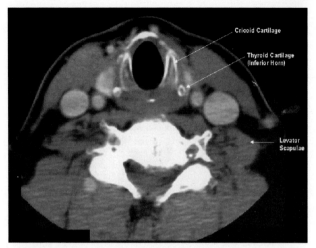

FIGURE 4.6: Axial CT section at the level of cricoid cartilage

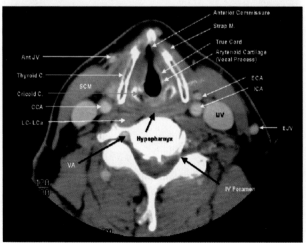

FIGURE 4.7: Axial CT section at the level of thyroid cartilage

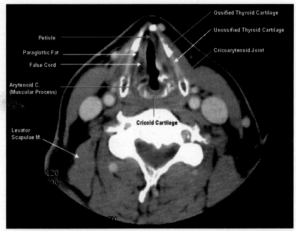

FIGURE 4.8: Axial CT section at the level of false cord

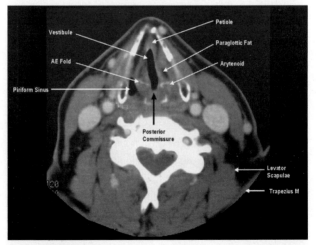

FIGURE 4.9: Axial CT section at the level of AE folds

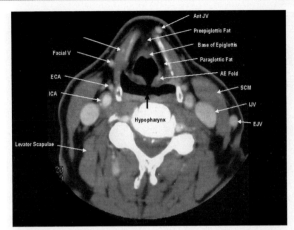

FIGURE 4.10: Axial CT section at the level of base of epiglottis

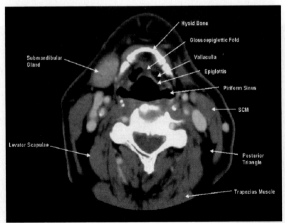

FIGURE 4.11: Axial CT section at the level of pyriform sinus

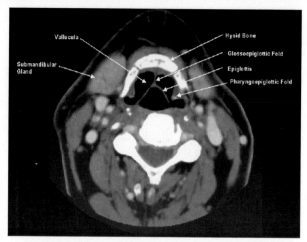

FIGURE 4.12: Axial CT section at the level of hyoid bone

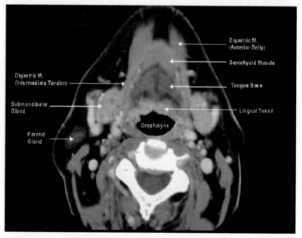

FIGURE 4.13: Axial CT section at the level of tongue base

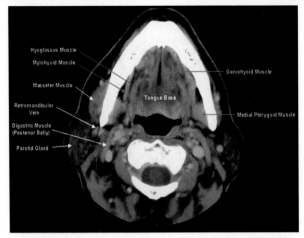

FIGURE 4.14: Axial CT section at the level of oropharynx

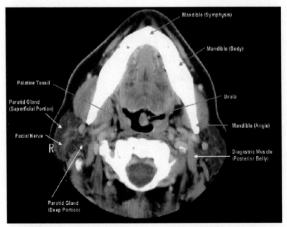

FIGURE 4.15: Axial CT section at the level of uvula

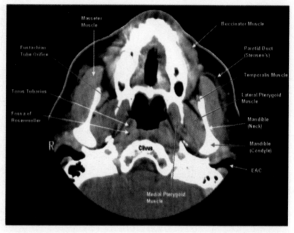

FIGURE 4.16: Axial CT section at the level of naxopharynx

NECK SPACES

Fascial layers of the neck are divided into
- Superficial cervical fascia (SCF)
- Deep cervical fascia (DCF)
- Superficial
- Middle layer (Visceral/pharyngomucosal)
- Deep (Prevertebral)

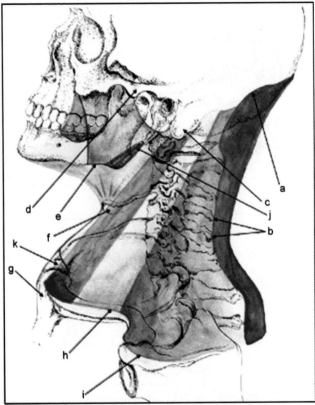

FIGURE 4.17: Investing layer of DCF

Superiorly
- Nuchal line of occipital bone (a)
- Spinous processes of cervical vertebrae & nuchal lig. (b)
- Mastoid processes (c)
- Zygomatic arches (d)
- Inferior border of mandible (e)
- Hyoid bone (f)

Inferiorly
- Manubrium (g)
- Clavicles (h)
- Acromion (i)

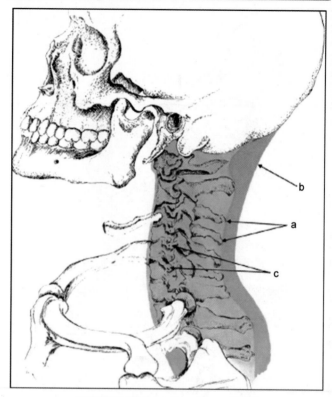

FIGURE 4.18: Prevertebral layer of DCF
- Superiorly—from base of skull
- Inferiorly—superior mediastinum
- Anteriorly—merges with the ALL up to T3-T4
- Posteriorly—from cervical spinous processes (a) and the ligamentum nuchae (b)

DCF—AXIAL PLANE

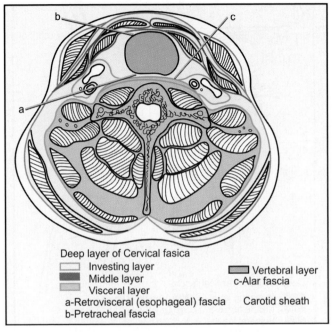

Deep layer of Cervical fasica

☐ Investing layer
■ Middle layer
☐ Visceral layer
a-Retrovisceral (esophageal) fascia
b-Pretracheal fascia

☐ Vertebral layer
c-Alar fascia

Carotid sheath

FIGURE 4.19: Deep cervical fascia—axial view

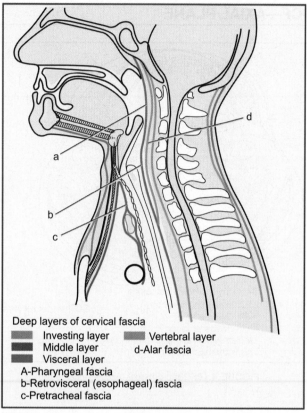

FIGURE 4.20: Diagram showing deep layers of cervical fascia—sagittal view

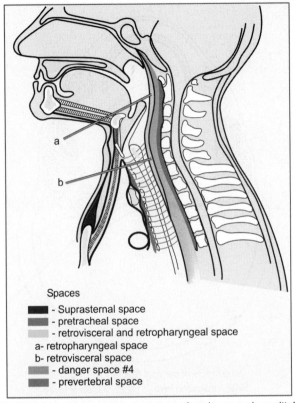

Spaces
- Suprasternal space
- pretracheal space
- retrovisceral and retropharyngeal space
a- retropharyngeal space
b- retrovisceral space
- danger space #4
- prevertebral space

FIGURE 4.21: Diagram showing extent of neck spaces in sagittal view

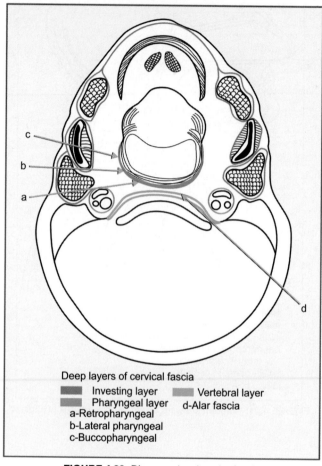

FIGURE 4.22: Diagram showing alar fascia

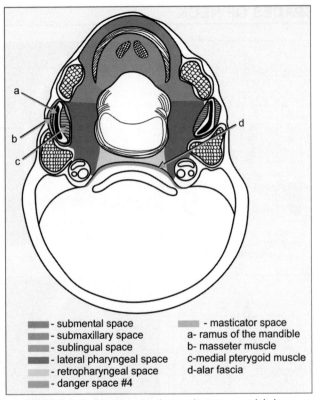

- submental space
- submaxillary space
- sublingual space
- lateral pharyngeal space
- retropharyngeal space
- danger space #4

- masticator space
a- ramus of the mandible
b- masseter muscle
c- medial pterygoid muscle
d- alar fascia

FIGURE 4.23: Diagram showing neck spaces—axial view

SPACES OF NECK

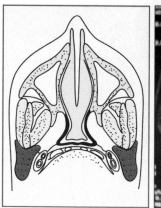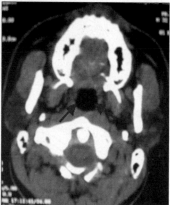

FIGURES 4.24A and B: Pharyngeal mucosa space

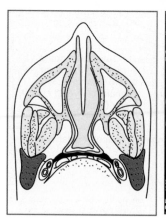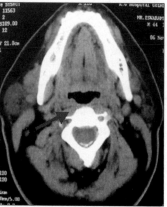

FIGURES 4.25A and B: Retropharyngeal space

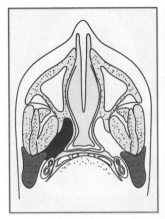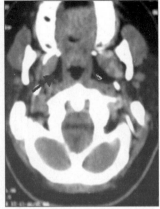

FIGURES 4.26A and B: Parapharyngeal space

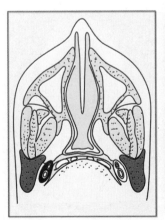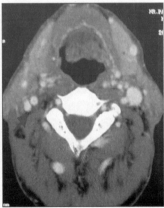

FIGURES 4.27A and B: Carotid space

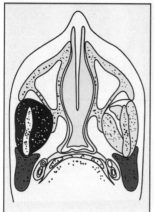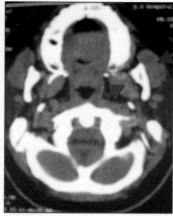

FIGURES 4.28A and B: Masticator space

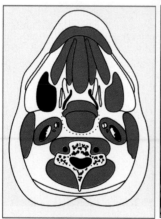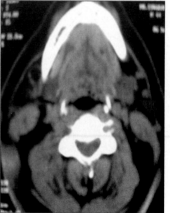

FIGURES 4.29A and B: Submandibular space

Chapter 5

Lungs

LUNGS

Organ	Location/Description	Notes
Pleura	Serous membrane lining the pleural cavity	There are two types of pleura: visceral pleura covers the lungs, parietal pleura lines the inner surfaces of the walls of pleural cavity; parietal pleura is sensitive to pain but visceral pleura is not sensitive to pain
Cervical parietal pleura	Serous membrane lining the pleural cavity which extends above the level of the 1st rib into the root of the neck	Cervical parietal pleura is continuous inferiorly with the costal and mediastinal parietal pleurae; it is reinforced by a specialization of scalene fascia (called Sibson's fascia or suprapleural membrane); also known as: cupula or cervical dome of pleura
Costal parietal pleura	Serous membrane lining the pleural cavity on the inner surfaces of the ribs, costal cartilages, and intercostal mm.	Costal parietal pleura is continuous anteriorly with the mediastinal parietal pleura at the costomediastinal reflection; it is continuous posteriorly with the mediastinal parietal pleural at the vertebral bodies; it is continuous inferiorly with the diaphragmatic parietal pleura at the costodiaphragmatic reflection; it is continuous superiorly with the cervical parietal pleura at the level of the 1st rib

Contd...

Contd...

Mediastinal parietal pleura	Serous membrane lining the pleural cavity on the lateral surface of the mediastinum	Mediastinal parietal pleura is continuous anteriorly with the costal parietal pleura at the costomediastinal reflection; it is continuous inferiorly with the diaphragmatic pleura at the inferomedial borders of the pleural cavities; it is continuous posteriorly with the costal parietal pleura lateral to the vertebral bodies; it is continuous superiorly with the cervical pleura at the level of the 1st rib
Visceral pleura	Serous membrane lining the surfaces of the lungs	Visceral pleura extends into the oblique and horizontal fissures of the lungs; it does not have pain fibers
Pulmonary ligament	Fold of pleura located below the root of the lung	Pulmonary ligament is where the visceral pleura and the mediastinal parietal pleura are continuous with each other
Cupula	Serous membrane lining the pleural cavity which extends above the level of the 1st rib into the root of the neck	Cupular pleura is continuous inferiorly with the costal and mediastinal parietal pleurae; it is reinforced by a specialization of scalene fascia (called Sibson's fascia or suprapleural membrane); also known as: cervical parietal pleura or cervical dome of pleura
Bronchi	The air conducting passages of the lungs	Bronchi may be classified as primary, secondary (lobar), and tertiary (segmental)
Primary bronchus	First branch of the air conducting system arising	Paired, right and left; one primary bronchus enters the

Contd...

Contd...

	from the bifurcation of the trachea at T4/T5 intervertebral disc	hilus of each lung; the right primary bronchus is shorter, larger in diameter and more vertically oriented than the left so that aspirated foreign bodies tend to lodge in the right primary bronchus
Secondary bronchus	A branch of the air conducting system arising from the primary bronchus	There are 3 secondary bronchi in the right lung: upper, middle, lower; there are 2 secondary bronchi in the left lung: upper, lower; also known as: lobar bronchi
Tertiary bronchus	A branch of the air conducting system arising from the secondary (lobar) bronchus	There are 10 tertiary bronchi in the right lung: branching from the right superior lobar bronchus—apical, anterior, posterior; branching from the right middle lobar bronchus—medial, lateral; branching from the right inferior lobar bronchus—superior, anterior basal, posterior basal, medial basal, lateral basal; there are 8 tertiary bronchi in the left lung: branching from the left superior lobar bronchus—apicoposterior, anterior; branching from the lingular bronchus (off of the superior lobar bronchus)—superior lingular, inferior lingular; branching from the inferior lobar bronchus—superior, anteromedial basal, posterior basal, lateral basal; also known as segmental bronchi

Contd...

Contd...

Segmental bronchus	A branch of the air conducting system arising from the secondary (lobar) bronchus	There are 10 tertiary bronchi in the right lung: branching from the right superior lobar bronchus—apical, anterior, posterior; branching from the right middle lobar bronchus—medial, lateral; branching from the right inferior lobar bronchus—superior, anterior basal, posterior basal, medial basal, lateral basal; there are 8 tertiary bronchi in the left lung: branching from the left superior lobar bronchus—apicoposterior, anterior; branching from the lingular bronchus (off of the superior lobar bronchus)—superior lingular, inferior lingular; branching from the inferior lobar bronchus—superior, anteromedial basal, posterior basal, lateral basal; also known as tertiary bronchi
Carina	Keel-shaped cartilage lying within the tracheal bifurcation	Carina trachealis is an important landmark during endoscopy of the bronchial tree
Lung	The portion of the respiratory system where exchange of gasses occurs between the air and the blood; located in the thoracic cavity	Paired; right lung is divided into three lobes: superior, middle and inferior; left lung has two lobes: superior and inferior

Contd...

Contd...

Oblique fissure	Deep groove in the surface of the lung that separates the upper lobe from the lower lobe (both lungs), and the middle lobe from the lower lobe (right lung)	Oblique fissure extends from the level of the T3 vertebra posteriorly to the 6th costo-chondral junction anteriorly
Horizontal fissure	Deep groove in the surface of the lung that separates the middle lobe from the upper lobe (right lung only)	Horizontal fissure extends from the 5th rib at the mid-axillary line along the 4th rib to the sternum anteriorly
Inferior lobe	The portion of the lung supplied by the inferior lobar bronchus	Inferior lobe of the right lung: possesses 5 bronchopulmonary segments—superior, anterior basal, posterior basal, medial basal, lateral basal; inferior lobe of the left lung: possesses 4 bronchopulmonary segments—superior, anteromedial basal, posterior basal, lateral basal
Middle lobe	The portion of the right lung supplied by the middle lobar bronchus	Middle lobe is found in the right lung only; it possesses 2 bronchopulmonary segments: medial and lateral; lingula of the inferior lobe of the left lung is equivalent to the middle lobe of the right lung
Superior lobe	The portion of the lung supplied by the superior lobar bronchus	Superior lobe of the right lung: possesses three bronchopulmonary segments—apical, anterior and posterior; superior lobe of the left lung: possesses four bronchopulmonary segments—apicoposterior, anterior, superior lingular, inferior lingular

ARTERIES

Artery	Source	Branches	Supply	Notes
Left bronchial	Descending thoracic aorta	Right bronchial a. (occasionally)	Lower trachea, bronchial tree	There are usually two left bronchial artery
Right bronchial	3rd right posterior intercostal	No named branches	Lower trachea, bronchial tree	Right bronchial artery may arise from the left bronchial artery
Pulmonary artery	Pulmonary trunk	Right: superior lobar a. to the superior lobe and inferior lobar a. to the middle and inferior lobes; left: superior lobar a. to the superior lobe, inferior lobar a. to the inferior lobe	Lungs	Each pulmonary artery carries deoxygenated blood to the hilum of one lung
Pulmonary trunk	Right ventricle	Right pulmonary artery, left pulmonary artery	Lungs	The pulmonary trunk carries de-oxygenated blood from the heart to the right and left pulmonary artery; each pulmonary artery carries deoxygenated blood to the hilum of one lung; bronchial aa. supply oxygenated blood to the tissues of the lung as far distally in the bronchial tree as the respiratory bronchioles

VEINS

Vein	Tributaries	Drains into	Region drained	Notes
Pulmonary	Lobar veins	Left atrium	Lungs	Usually two pulmonary veins per side, superior and inferior; all empty into the left atrium

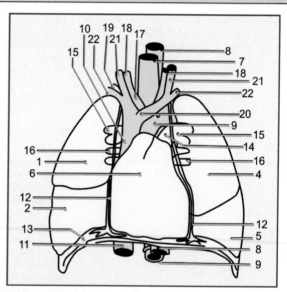

FIGURE 5.1: Anterior view of heart and lungs. (1) Upper lobe of right lung, (2) Middle lobe of right lung, (3) Lower lobe of right lung, (4) Upper lobe of left lung, (5) Lower lobe of left lung, (6) Heart in pericardial sac, (7) Trachea, (8) Oesophagus, (9) Aorta, (10) Superior vena cava, (11) Inferior vena cava, (12) Phrenic nerve, (13) Diaphragm, (14) Pulmonary trunk, (15) Pulmonary arteries, (16) Pulmonary veins, (17) Brachiocephalic trunk, (18) Common carotid arteries, (19) Subclavian arteries, (20) Innominate veins, (21) Internal jugular veins, (22) Subclavian veins

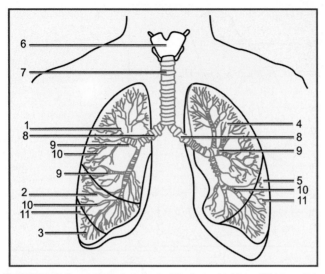

FIGURE 5.2: General arrangement of the bronchial tree. (1) Upper lobe of right lung, (2) Middle lobe of right lung, (3) Lower lobe of right lung, (4) Upper lobe of left lung, (5) Lower lobe of left lung, (6) Pharynx, (7) Trachea, (8) Principle bronchi, (9) Lobar bronchi, (10) Segmental bronchi, (11) Bronchioles

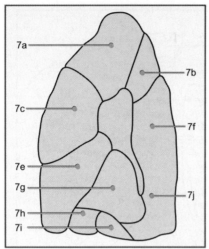

FIG. 5.3

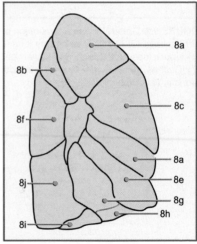

FIGURES 5.3 and 5.4:: (A) Right lung—medial view, (B) Left lung—medial view (For legends see Figure 5.6)

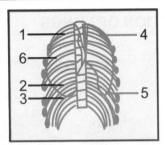

FIGURE 5.5: Lungs-anterior view, (1) Upper lobe of right lung, (2) Middle lobe of right lung, (3) Lower lobe of right lung, (4) upper lobe of left lung, (5) Lower lobe of left lung, (6) Interlobar fissures

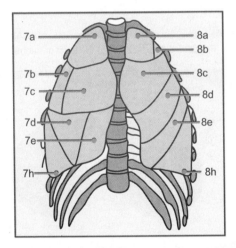

FIGURE 5.6: Segments of right lung. (7a) Apical, (7b) Posterior, (7c) Anterior, (7d) Lateral, (7e) Medial, (7f) Superior (apical), (7g) Medial basal, (7h) Anterior basal, (7i) Lateral basal, (7j) Posterior basal, (8) Segments of left lung, (8a) Apical, (8b) Posterior, (8c) Anterior, (8d) Superior lingular, (8e) Inferior lingular, (8f) Superior (apical), (8g) Medial basal, (8h) Anterior basal, (8i) Lateral basal, (8j) Posterior basal

AXIAL SECTION OF LUNGS

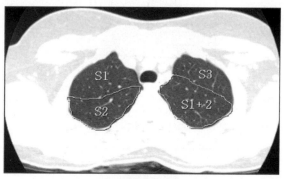

FIGURE 5.7A: Axial CT at the level of trachea

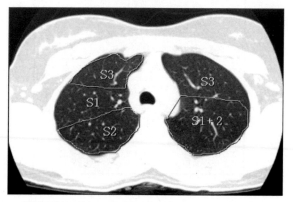

FIGURE 5.7B: Axial CT at the level of arch of aorta

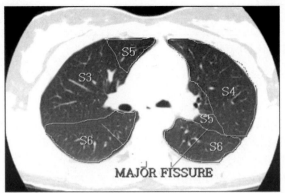

FIGURE 5.8A: Axial CT at the level of carina

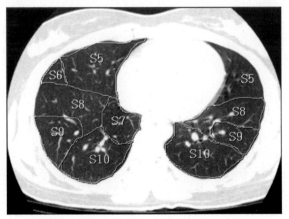

FIGURE 5.8B: Axial CT at the level of ventricles

	Segment	Bronchus
Right Upper Lobe		
Apical	S1	B1
Posterior	S2	B2
Anterior	S3	B3
Right Middle Lobe		
Lateral	S4	B4
Medial	S5	B5
Right Lower Lobe		
Superior	S6	B6
Medial basal	S7	B7
Anterior basal	S8	B8
Lateral basal	S9	B9
Posterior basal	S10	B10
Left Upper Lobe		
Apical posterior	S1+2	B1+2
Anterior	S3	B3
Superior lingular	S4	B4
Inferior lingular	S5	B5
Left Lower Lobe		
Superior	S6	B6
Anterior medial basal	S8	B8
Lateral basal	S9	B9
Posterior basal	S10	B10

FISSURAL ANATOMY OF LUNGS

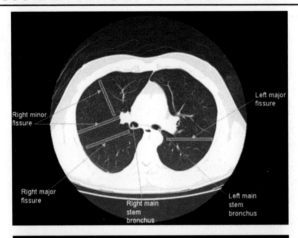

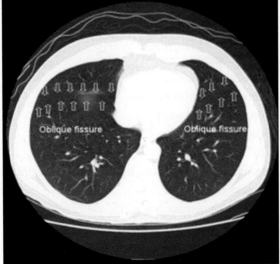

FIGURES 5.9A and B: Axial CT showing position of fissures of lung

MEDIASTINUM AXIAL VIEWS

See Figures 5.10 to 5.18.

These are axial views of the chest with emphasis on the mediastinum as seen by Computed Tomography. Structures to be identified are:

1. Trachea
2. Esophagus
3. Trapezius muscle
4. Clavicle
5. Subscapularis muscle
6. Infraspinatus muscle
7. Supraspinatus muscle
8. Pectoralis major muscle
9. Pectoralis minor muscle
10. Serratus anterior muscle
11. Latissimus dorsi muscle
12. Erector spinae muscles
13. Subclavian arteries
14. Common carotid arteries
15. Internal jugular veins
16. Scapula
17. Rib
18. Manubrium of sternum, body of sternum xiphoid—process of sternum
19. Aortic arch, ascending aorta, descending aorta
20. Azygous vein, arch of the azygous
21. Brachiocephalic veins
22. Superior vena cava

23. Thymus gland
24. Teres major muscle
25. Teres minor muscle
26. Left subclavian vein/axillary vein
27. Brachiocephalic artery
28. Inferior vena cava
29. Pulmonary trunk
30. Pulmonary arteries
31. Thoracic duct
32. Carina of trachea
33. Right ventricle
34. Right atrium
35. Left atrium
36. Left ventricle
37. Pulmonary vein
38. Interventricular septum
39. Coronary sinus

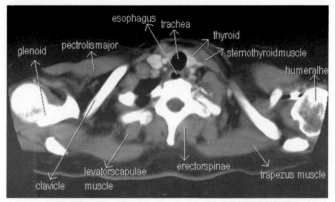

FIGURE 5.10: Axial section at the level of the trachea

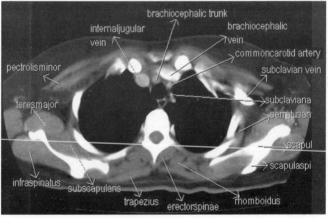

FIGURE 5.11: Axial section at the level of brachicephalic vessels

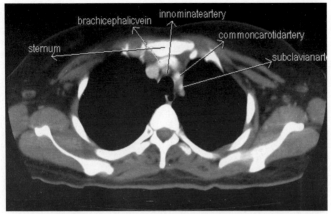

FIGURE 5.12: Axial CT at the level of SVC formation

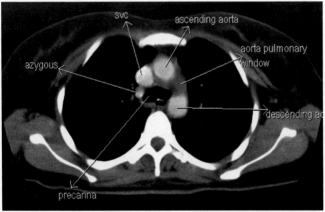

FIGURE 5.13: Axial CT at the level of AP window

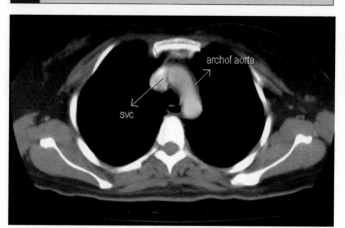

FIGURE 5.14: Axial CT at the level of arch of aorta

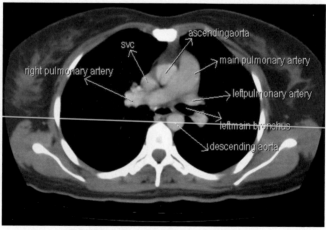

FIGURE 5.15: Axial CT at the level of MPA

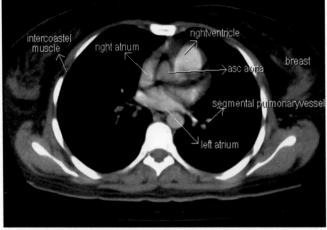

FIGURE 5.16: Axial CT at the artrial level

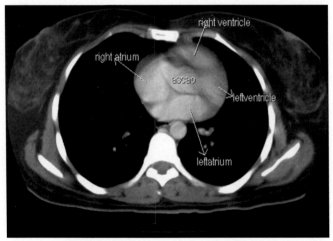

FIGURE 5.17: Axial CT at the ventricular level

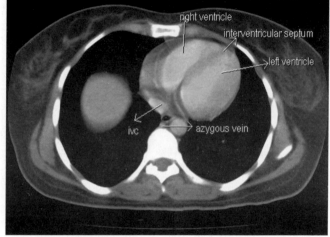

FIGURE 5.18: Axial CT at the level of diaphragmatic dome

Chapter 6

Abdomen

AXIAL ANATOMY— ABDOMEN

Structure to be identified
1) Liver, (2) Spleen, (3) Pancreas, (4) Gallbladder, (5) Right adrenal gland, (6) Adrenal glands, (7) Inferior vena cava, (8) Aorta, (9) Portal vein, (10) Superior mesenteric artery, (10*) Superior mesenteric vein, (11) Ascending, (12) Descending colon, (13) Transverse colon, (14) Stomach, (15) Duodenum, (16) Right kidney, (17) Left kidney, (18) Inferior mesenteric artery, (19) Duodenum, 2nd part, (19*) Duodenum, 3rd part, (20) Left renal vein, (20*) Left renal artery, (21) Right renal vein, (21*) Right renal artery, (22) Small intestine, (23) Splenic artery, (24) Celiac trunk, (25) Splenic vein, (26) Anterior and posterior abdominal wall muscles.

PELVIS AND UPPER THIGH

Structure to be identified
(1) Aorta, (2) Inferior vena cava, (3) Ureter, (5) Small bowel, (6) Cecum appendix 7) Descending colon, (8) Psoas muscle, (9) Erector spinae muscle, (10) Rectus abdominus muscle, (11) External oblique muscle, (12) Internal oblique muscle, (13) Tranversus abdominus muscle, (14) Quadratus lumborum muscle, (15) Vertebra, (body), (16) Vertebra (spinous process), (17) Common iliac arteries, (17a) Common iliac veins, (18) Iliac wing, (19) External iliac vessels, (20) Common femoral artery and vein, (21) Superficial femoral artery, (22) Deep femoral artery, (23) Iliacus muscle, (24) Gluteus maximus

muscle, (25) Gluteus medius muscle, (26) Gluteus minimus muscle, (27) Sacrum, (28) Urinary bladder, (29) Sigmoid colon, (30) Rectum, (31) Seminal vesicle, (32) Prostate gland, (33) Base of penis, (34) Piriformis muscle, (35) Ischial spine, (36) Femoral head, (37) Greater trochanter, (38) Rectus femoris muscle, (39) Internal obturator muscle, (40) External obturator muscle, (41) Ischiorectal fossa, (42) Symphysis pubis, (43) Inferior pubic ramus, (44) Ischial ruberosity, (45) Gracilis muscle, (46) Sartorius muscle, (47) Adductor magnus muscle, (48) Adductor longus muscle 49) Vastus lateralis muscle, (50) Vastus intermedius muscle, (51) Vastus medialis muscle, (52) Semimembranousus and semitendinosus muscles, (54) Tensor fascia latae, (55) Pectineus muscle.

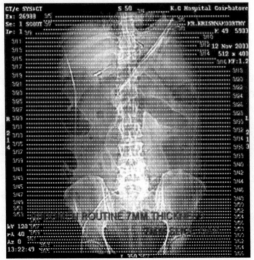

FIGURE 6.1A: Digital scanogram for planning axial slices

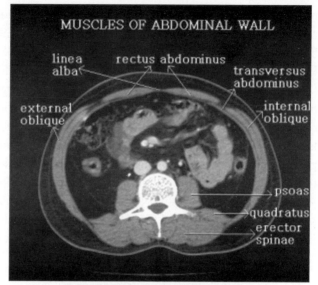

FIGURE 6.1B: Axial CT sections showing abdominal wall muscles

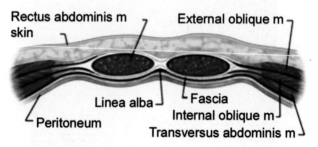

FIGURE 6.2: Schematic for anterior abdominal wall muscle planes

LIVER SEGMENTS

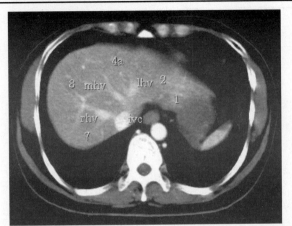

FIGURE 6.3: Axial CT at the level of hepatic vein confluence. RhV—Right hepatic vein, MhV—Middle hepatic vein; LHV—Left hepatic vein. IVC—Inferior vena cava

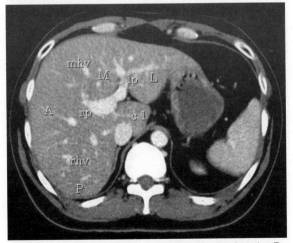

FIGURE 6.4: Axial CT at level of caudate lobe. A—Anterior, P—Posterior, M—Medial, L—Lateral segments

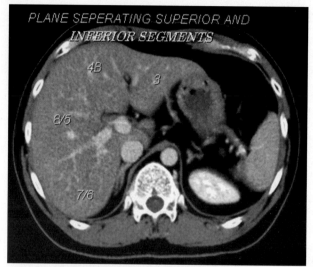

FIGURE 6.5: Axial CT at the level of porta

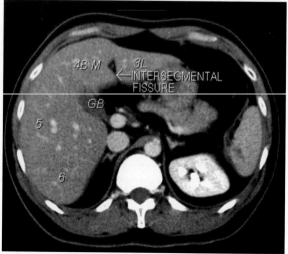

FIGURE 6.6: Axial CT at the level of GB

SURFACE REFORMATION

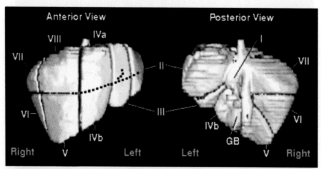

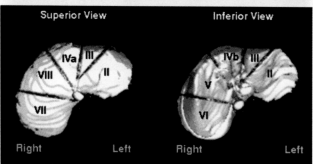

FIGURES 6.7A and B: Surface rendering of liver segments

I.	caudate
II.	left posterolateral segment
III.	left anterolateral segment
IVa.	left superomedial segment
IVb.	left inferomedial segment
V.	right anteroinferior segment
VI.	right posteroinferior segment
VII.	right posterosuperior segment
VIII.	right anterosuperior segment

SEGMENTS OF LIVER

PANCREAS

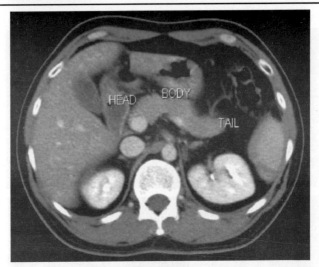

FIGURE 6.8: Axial CT of pancreas

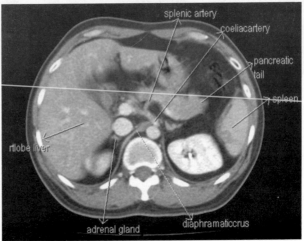

FIGURE 6.9: Axial section at the celiac axis level

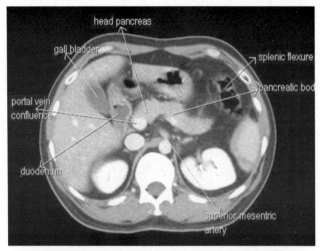

FIGURE 6.10: Axial sections at the level of SMA

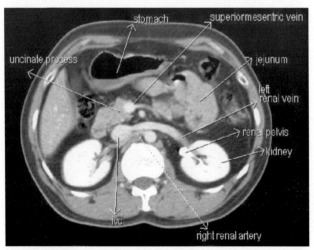

FIGURE 6.11: Axial sections at the level of renal hilum

INTRAHEPATIC BILE DUCTS

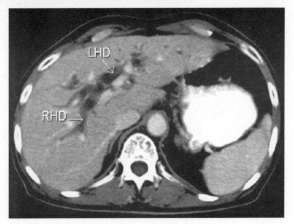

FIGURE 6.12: Axial CT showing dilated right and left hepatic ducts

DOUBLE DUCTS PD, CBD

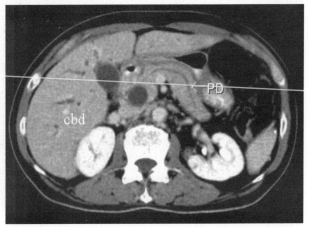

FIGURE 6.13: Axial CT showing dilated CBD and pancreatic duct

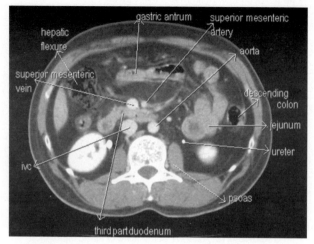

FIGURE 6.14: Axial CT at the level of third part of duodenum

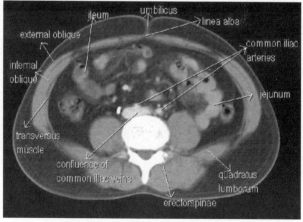

FIGURE 6.15: Axial CT at the level of IVC origin

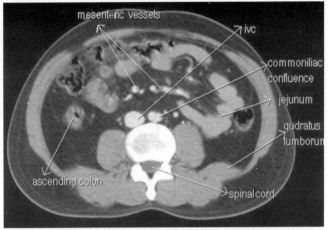

FIGURE 6.16: Axial CT at the level of aortic bifurcation

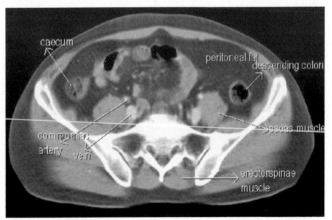

FIGURE 6.17: Axial CT at the level of caecum

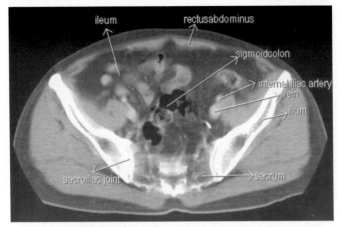

FIGURE 6.18: Axial CT at the level of sigmoid colon

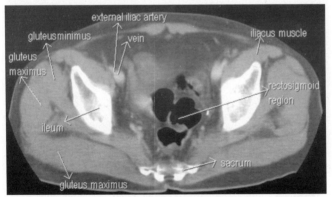

FIGURE 6.19: Axial CT at the level of rectosegmoid junction

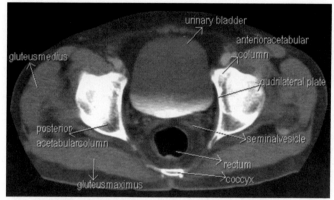

FIGURE 6.20: Axial CT at the level of urinary bladder

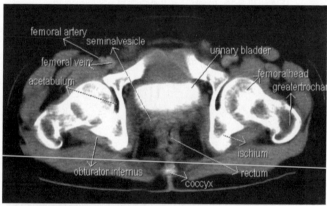

FIGURE 6.21: Axial CT at the level of pubic symphysis

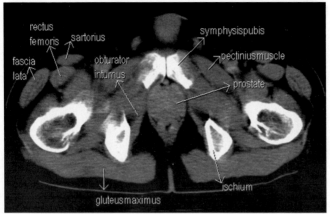

FIGURE 6.22: Axial CT at the level of ischium

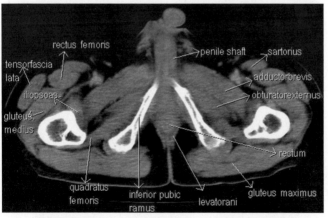

FIGURE 6.23: Axial CT at the level of inferior pubic ramus

UTERUS AND OVARIES

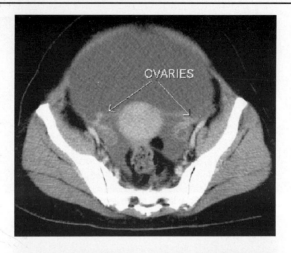

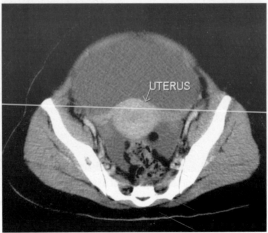

FIGURES 6.24A and B: Axial CT in a Patients with ascites showing ovaries and uterus

MUSCLES AND PELVIC STRUCTURES

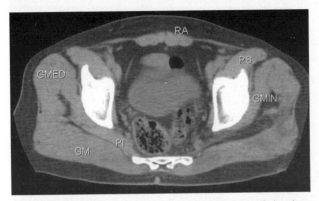

FIGURE 6.25: Axial CT at the level of acetabular roof showing
muscles of pelvis

RA—Rectus Abdominis	PS—Psoa S
GMIN—Gluteus Minimus	GMED—Gluteus Medius
GM—Gluteus Maximus	PI—Piriformis

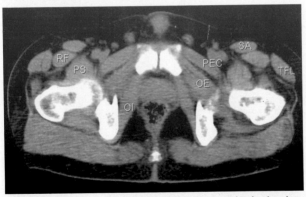

FIGURE 6.26: Axial CT at the level of pubic symphysis showing
muscles

OI—Obturator Internus	OE—Obturator Externus
PEC—Pectineus	SA—Sartorius
PS—Psoa S	EF—Rectus Femoris

INDIVIDUAL BOWEL PATTERNS

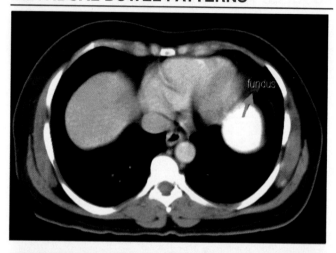

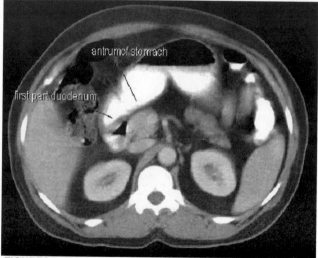

FIGURES 6.27A and B: Axial CT showing the fundus and antrum of stomach

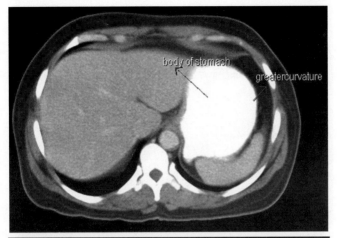

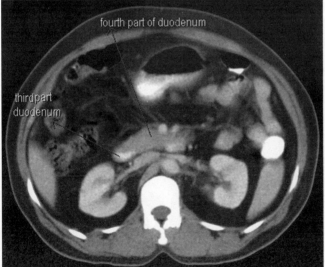

FIGURES 6.28A and B: Axial CT showing the body of stomach and third, fourth part of duodenum

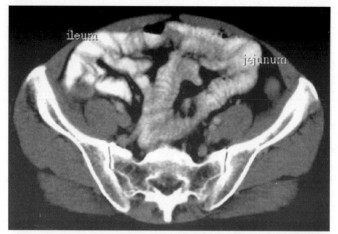

FIGURE 6.29: Axial CT showing the jejunal and ileal bowel patterns

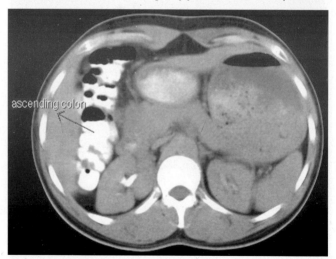

FIGURE 6.30: Axial CT showing the ascending colon

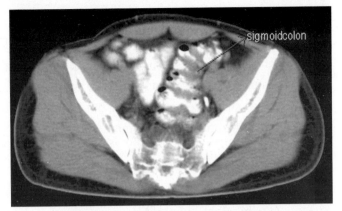

FIGURE 6.31: Axial CT showing the sigmoid colon

CT PERITONEOGRAM—SHOWING PERITONEAL SPACES

PERITONEAL SPACES

The peritoneal cavity is divided into two main compartments, the supramesocolic and the inframesocolic, by the transverse colon and its mesentery connecting it to the posterior abdominal wall The root of the transverse mesocolon subextends across the infra-ampullary segment of the descending duodenum, the head of the pancreas, and continues along the lower edge of the body and tail of the pancreas.

The Supramesocolic Compartment

The supramesocolic compartment can be arbitrarily divided into right and left supramesocolic peritoneal spaces. These regions can also be divided into a number of subspaces, which are normally in communication, but often become separated by inflammatory membranes in disease.

Right Supramesocolic Space

The right supramesocolic space has three subextends spaces: (a) the right subphrenic space; (b) the right subhepatic space, which can be further divided arbitrarily into anterior and posterior areas; and (c) the lesser sac. The right subphrenic space extends over the diaphragmatic surface of the right lobe of the liver to the right coronary ligament posteroinferiorly and the falciform ligament medially, which separates it from the left subphrenic space In the presence of infected fluid, pyogenic membranes may divide the right subphrenic space into anterior and posterior compartments.

The right subhepatic space can be arbitrarily divided into anterior and posterior spaces. The anterior right subhepatic space is limited inferiorly by the transverse colon and its mesentery. The posterior right subhepatic space, also known as the hepatorenal fossa or Morison's pouch, extends posteriorly to the parietal peritoneum overlying the right

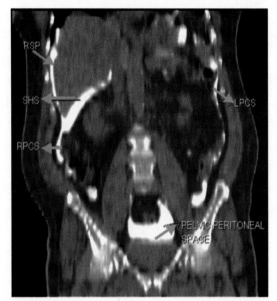

FIGURE 6.32: Coronal CT reformation after CT peritoneogram revealing the peritoneal spaces. RSP—Right subphrenic space, SHS—Right subhepatic space, RPCS—Right paracolic space, LPCS—Left paracolic space

kidney. Superiorly the right subhepatic space is bounded by the inferior surface of the right lobe of the liver.

It communicates freely with the right subphrenic space and the right paracolic gutter. In the supine patient, the posterior right subhepatic space (the hepatorenal fossa or Morison's pouch) is more dependent than the right paracolic gutter, and thus under the force of gravity, fluid collections are common in this location.

The lesser sac extends to the left, behind the stomach and anterior to the pancreas It is considered to be part of the right supramesocolic space, as embryologically the growth of the liver into the right peritoneal space stretches the dorsal mesentery and forms the future lesser sac posterior to the stomach. It communicates with the rest of the peritoneal cavity through a narrow inlet, the epiploic foramen (foramen of Winslow), between the inferior vena cava and the free margin of the hepatoduodenal ligament. The lesser sac lies posterior to the lesser omentum, stomach, duodenal bulb and gastrocolic ligament.

A prominent oblique fold of peritoneum is raised on the posterior wall of the lesser sac by the left gastric artery, dividing it into two major recesses. The smaller superior recess completely encloses the caudate lobe of the liver. At the porta hepatis this recess lies posterior to the portal vein. Superiorly it extends deep into the fissure for the ligamentum venosum and posteriorly lies adjacent to the right diaphragmatic crus. The larger inferior recess lies between the stomach and the pancreas. It is bounded inferiorly by the transverse colon and its mesentery, but can extend for a variable distance between the leaves of the greater omentum. To the left it is bounded by the gastrosplenic and splenorenal ligaments which meet at the splenic hilum.

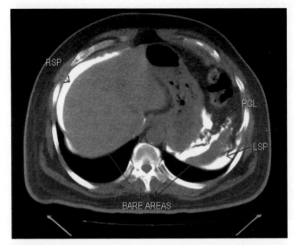

FIGURE 6.33: CT peritoneuogram showing right subphrenic space (RSP), Left subphrenic space (LSP), phrenico colic ligament (PCL)

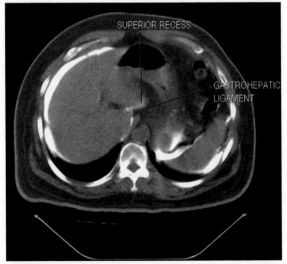

FIGURE 6.34: CT peritoneogram showing superior recess of lesser sac

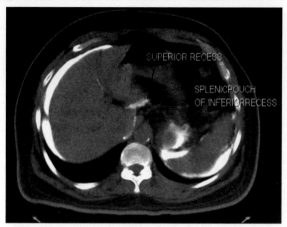

FIGURE 6.35: CT peritoneogram showing pouch of inferior recess

Left Supramesocolic Space

The left supramesocolic space has four arbitrary subspaces, which are in communication in normal anatomy : (a) the anterior left peri-hepatic space; (b) the posterior left perihepatic space, surrounding the lateral segment of the left hepatic lobe; (c) the anterior left subphrenic spaces;and (d) the posterior left subphrenic (perisplenic) space, superior to gastric fundus and spleen.

The left anterior perihepatic space is bounded medially by the falciform ligament, posteriorly by the liver surface and left coronary ligament, and anteriorly by the diaphragm. It communicates superiorly and to the left with The left anterior perihepatic space is bounded medially by the falciform ligament, posteriorly by the liver surface and left coronary ligament, and anteriorly by the diaphragm. It communicates superiorly and to the left with the left anterior subphrenic space, and inferiorly with the greater peritoneal cavity over the surface of the transverse mesocolon.

The Inframesocolic Compartment

The inframesocolic compartment is divided into two unequal spaces posteriorly by the root of the small bowel mesentery, as this runs from the duodenojejunal flexure in the left upper quadrant to the ileocaecal valve in the right lower quadrant. It also contains the right and left paratherecolic gutters lateral to the ascending and descending colon.

The Right Inframesocolic Space

This triangular space is smaller than its counter-part on the left. It is bounded by the transverse surcolon superiorly and to the right, and by the root of the small bowel mesentery, as this runs from the duodenojejunal flexure to the ileocaecal junction inferiorly and to the left.

The Left Inframesocolic Space

This space is larger than its counterpart on the right and is in free communication with the pelvis on the right of the midline. The sigmoid colon and its associated mesentery form a partial barrier on the left of the midline.

The Paracolic Gutters

These are the peritoneal recesses on the posterior gastro-abdominal wall lateral to the ascending and descending colon. The right paracolic gutter is continuous superiorly with the right subhepatic and subphrenic spaces. It is larger than the left paracolic gutter, which is partially separated from the left subphrenic spaces by the phrenicocolic ligament. Both paracolic spaces are in continuity with the pelvic peritoneal spaces.

The Pelvic Peritoneal Spaces

Inferiorly the peritoneum is reflected over the fundus of the bladder, the anterior and posterior surface of the uterus and upper posterior vagina in females, and on to the front of the rectum at the junction of its middle and lower thirds. The urinary bladder subdivides the pelvis into right and left paravesical spaces. In men parathere is only one potential space for fluid collection posterior to the bladder, the rectovesical pouch.

In women there are two potential spaces posterior to the bladder, the uterovesical pouch, and posterior to the uterus the deeper rectouterine pouch (pouch of Douglas) The layers of peritoneum on the anterior and posterior surcolon faces of the uterus are reflected laterally to the pelvic side walls as the broad ligaments, containing the uterine (Fallopian) tubes.

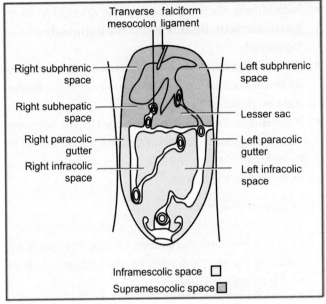

FIGURE 6.36: Schematic diagram of peritoneal space

Omentum

- This is a **double-layered sheet or fold of peritoneum**.
- The lesser and greater omentum attach the stomach to the body wall or to other abdominal organs.

The Lesser Omentum

- This fold of peritoneum connects the **lesser curvature of the stomach** and the **proximal part of the duodenum** to the **liver**.

- Individually, these connections are referred to as the **gastrohepatic ligament** and the **hepatoduodenal ligament**.
- The lesser omentum lies **posterior to the left lobe of the liver** and is attached to the liver in the **fissure for the ligamentum venosum**.
- It is also attached to the **porta hepatis**, the transverse fissure or gate *(L. porta)* on the inferior surface of the liver through which the bile duct, vessels, and nerves enter or leave the liver.

The Greater Omentum

- This is a fat-laden fold of peritoneum that hangs down from the **greater curvature of the stomach** and connects the stomach with the **diaphragm**, **spleen**, and **transverse colon**.
- This double-layered peritoneal fold normally fuses during the foetal period, thereby **obliterating the inferior recess of the omental bursa**.
- As a result, the apron-like greater omentum is **composed of four layers of peritoneum**.
- After passing inferiorly as far as the pelvis, the greater omentum **loops back on itself**, overlying and **attaching to the transverse colon**.

Peritoneal Ligaments

- A peritoneal ligament is a **double layer of peritoneum** that connects an organ with another organ or with the abdominal wall.

- Ligaments may contain blood vessels or remnants of vessels (e.g. the falciform ligament contains the ligamentum teres, a remnant of the fetal umbilical vein).
- The greater omentum is divided into **3 parts**:
  1. The apron-like part, called the **gastrocolic ligament**, is attached to the **transverse colon**.
  2. The left part, called the **gastrosplenic ligament** (gastrolienal ligament), connects the hilum of the spleen to the greater curvature and fundus of the stomach.
  3. The superior part called the **gastrophrenic ligament** is attached to the diaphragm and the posterior aspect of the fundus and the oesophagus.
- The **falciform ligament** extends from the liver to the anterior abdominal wall and the diaphragm.
- The **ligamentum teres** is the obliterated remnant of the **left umbilical vein**, lying in the free edge of the falciform ligament and extending from the groove for the ligamentum teres to the umbilicus.
- The **superior (anterior) and inferior (posterior) layers of the coronary ligament** are reflections of the peritoneum, which surround the bare area of the liver.
- The **left and right triangular ligaments** are where the layers of the coronary ligament meet to the left and right respectively.
- The falciform, coronary and triangular ligaments are **derived from** that part of the **ventral mesogastrium connecting the liver to the body wall**.

- The gastrohepatic and hepatoduodenal ligaments are **derived from** that part of the **ventral mesogastrium connecting the stomach and the liver**.
- The gastrosplenic and gastrophrenic, as well as the lienorenal and phrenicolienal ligaments are **derived from the dorsal mesogastrium**.

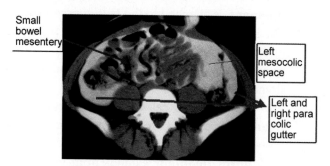

FIGURE 6.37: CT peritoneogram showing folds of mesentery

The Peritoneal Folds

- A peritoneal fold (*L. plica*) is a reflection of peritoneum with more or less sharp borders.
- Often it is formed by peritoneum that covers blood vessels, ducts, and obliterated fetal vessels.
- Several folds are visible on the **parietal peritoneum** on the **interior** of the anterior abdominal wall.
- The **median umbilical fold** contains the **urachus**, which extends from the urinary bladder to the umbilicus.

- The **medial umbilical folds** are raised by the obliterated umbilical arteries, extending from the internal iliac arteries to the umbilicus.
- The **lateral umbilical folds** are raised by the inferior epigastric arteries, extending from the deep inguinal rings on each side to the arcuate lines.

Peritoneal Pouches

- The **rectouterine pouch** (in females) separating the rectus from the bladder.
- The **rectovesical pouch** (in males) separating the rectum from the bladder.
- The **vesicounterine pouch** (in females) separating the bladder from the uterus

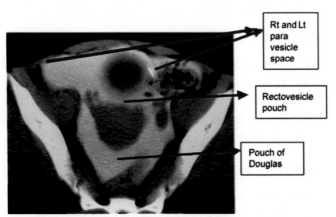

FIGURE 6.38: CT peritoneogram showing pelvic spaces

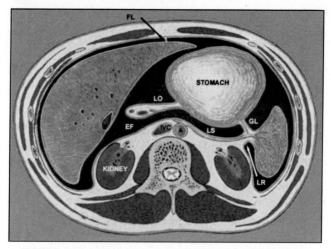

FIGURE 6.39: Schematic diagram showing perigastric ligaments
- falciform ligament FL
- gastrolienal ligament GL
- lienorenal ligament LR
- lesser omentum LO

RETROPERITONEUM

Extraperitoneal space is divided in to the anterior and posterior pararenal space and the perinephric space by the anterior and posterior layers of the renal fascia. Both these fascia fuse to form the lateral conal fascia behind the descending colon.

ANTERIOR PARARENAL COMPARTMENT

The anterior pararenal compartment lies between the anterior renal fascia and the posterior parietal peritoneum. The lateral border is defined by the lateroconal fascia and the compartment is potentially contiguous across the midline. Contents include pancreas, the descending, horizontal and terminal portions of duodenum. The ascending and descending colon.

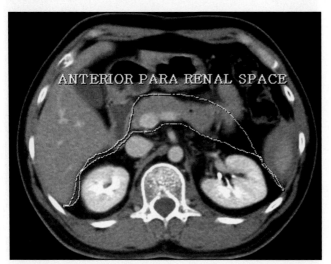

FIGURE 6.40: Anterior pararenal space

PERINEPHRIC COMPARTMENT

Formed by fusion of the anterior (gerotas) and posterior (zuckercandles) fascia superiorly it fuses with the diaphragmatic fascia and laterally with the lateroconal fascia.

The inferior portion of the space is open towards the iliac fossa medially the posterior renal fascia fuses with the quadratus and psoas fascia.

Contents include adrenals, kidneys, renal vasculature, proximal part of renal collecting system.

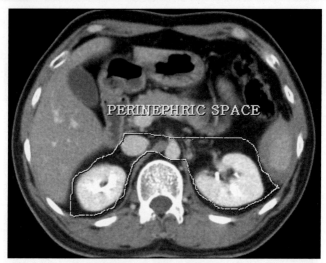

FIGURE 6.41: Perinephric space

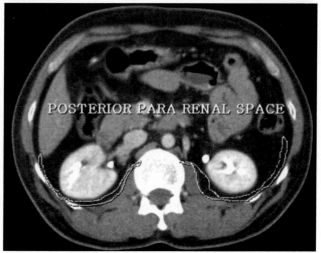

FIGURE 6.42: Posterior pararenal space

POSTERIOR PARARENAL COMPARTMENT

Lies between the posterior renal fascia and the transversalis fascia, it contains fat tissue and continues laterally as the propertoneal fat. The space is open inferiorly at the iliac crest. Medially the space is contained by the fusion of the transversallis and psoas fascias.

Chapter 7

Lower Limb

ANKLE JOINT (ANTEROPOSTERIOR)

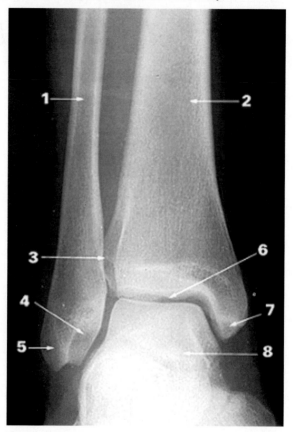

FIGURE 7.1: Ankle joint (Anteroposterior). (1) Fibula, (2) Tibia, (3) Distal tibiofibular joint, (4) Malleolar fossa, (5) Lateral malleolus, (6) Ankle joint, (7) Medial malleolus, (8) Talus

ANKLE JOINT (LATERAL)

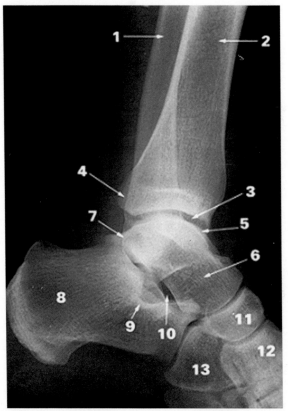

FIGURE 7.2: Ankle joint (lateral) (1) Fibula, (2) Tibia, (3) Ankle joint, (4) Promontory of tibia, (5) Trochlear surface of talus, (6) Talus, (7) Posterior tubercle of talus, (8) Calcaneus, (9) Sustentaculum tali, (10) Tarsal tunnel, (11) Navicular, (12) Cuneiforms, (13) Cuboid

FOOT (DORSO-PLANTAR)

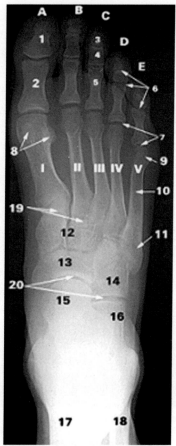

FIGURE 7.3: Foot (Dorso-plantar) (1,3) Distal phalax, (4) Middle phalax, (2,5) Proximal phalax, (6) Interphalangeal joints, (7) Metatarsophalangeal joints, (8) Sesamoids, (9) Head of metatarsal, (10) Shaft (body) of metatarsal, (11) Base of metatarsal, (12) Cuneiforms, (13) Navicular, (14) Cuboid, (15) Talus, (16) Calcaneus, (17) Tibia, (18) Fibula, (19) Tarsometatarsal joints, (20) Transverse midtarsal joint

HIP JOINT (ANTEROPOSTERIOR)

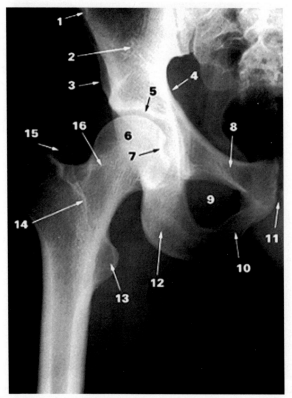

FIGURE 7.4: Hip joint (Anteroposterior). (1) Anterior superior iliac spine, (2) Ilium, (3) Anterior inferior iliac spine, (4) Pelvic brim, (5) Acetabular fossa, (6) Head of femur, (7) Fovea, (8) Superior ramus of pubis, (9) Obturator foramen, (10) Inferior ramus of pubis, (11) Pubic symphysis, (12) Ischium, (13) Lesser trochanter, (14) Intertrochanteric crest, (15) Greater trochanter, (16) Neck of femur

KNEE JOINT (LATERAL)

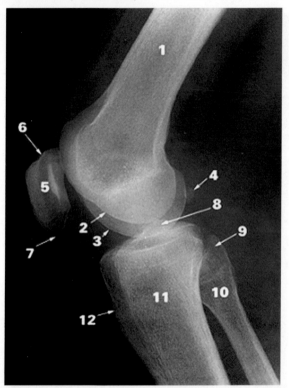

FIGURE 7.5: Knee joint (lateral). (1) Femur, (2) Lateral condyle of femur, (3) Medial condyle of femur, (4) Fabella, (5) Patella, (6) Base of patella, (7) Apex of patella, (8) Intercondylar eminence, (9) Apex of fibula, (10) Fibula, (11) Tibia, (12) Tibial tuberosity

OSTEOLOGY

Bone	Structure	Description
Tibia		The bone on the medial side of the leg
	Medial condyle	The heavy prominence on the medial side of the proximal end of the tibia
	Lateral condyle	The heavy prominence on the lateral side of the proximal end of the tibia
	Intercondylar eminence	The ridge of bone on the proximal end of the tibia that projects between the condyles
	Tibial tuberosity	The roughened protuberance on the anterior surface of the tibia located just distal to the condyles
	Body	The long, robust shaft of the tibia
	Interosseous border	The sharp ridge that runs longitudinally along the junction of the lateral surface and the posterior surface of the tibia
	Soleal line	A ridge of bone that descends obliquely from lateral to medial on the posterior surface of the tibia
	Medial malleolus	The large bony prominence on the medial side of the ankle
Fibula		The slender bone on the lateral side of the leg
	Head	The enlarged proximal end of the fibula
	Neck	The constricted portion of the fibula located just inferior to the head
	Body	The long slender shaft of the fibula
	Interosseous border	The sharp ridge that runs longitudinally along the medial surface of the fibula
	Lateral malleolus	The enlarged distal end of the fibula
Tarsal bones		The bones of the ankle
Talus		The most proximal of the tarsal bones
	Body	The proximal part of the talus
	Trochlea	The superior portion of the body of the talus that lies between the two malleoli
	Head	The portion of the talus that projects anteriorly

Contd...

Contd...

	Neck	The constricted part of the talus located proximal to the head
Calcaneus		The tarsal bone which forms the heel
	Calcaneal tuberosity	The posterior roughened area of the calcaneus which contacts the ground during weight-bearing
	Sustentaculum tali	The shelf-like medial projection of bone located inferior to the medial malleolus
Navicular		The tarsal bone located distal to the talus and proximal to the three cuneiform bones
Cuneiform, Medial		The most medial bone in the distal row of tarsal bones
Cuneiform, Middle		The intermediate bone of the three cuneiform bones
Cuneiform, Lateral		The bone that is located between the middle cuneiform and the cuboid bone
Cuboid		The most lateral bone in the distal row of tarsal bones
Metatarsals		The bones located between the tarsal bones and the phalanges
	Base	The proximal end of the metatarsal
	Body	The slender shaft of the metatarsal
	Head	The rounded distal end of the metatarsal
Phalanx (phalanges)		The distal two or three bones in the digits of the foot
	Base	The proximal end of the phalanx
	Body	The slender shaft of the phalanx
	Head	The distal end of the phalanx

MUSCLES

Muscle	Origin	Insertion
Extensor digitorum brevis	Superolateral surface of the calcaneus	Extensor expansion of toes 1-4
Extensor digitorum longus	Lateral condyle of the tibia, anterior surface of the fibula, lateral portion of the interosseous membrane	Dorsum of the lateral 4 toes via extensor expansions (central slip inserts on base of middle phalanx, lateral slips on base of distal phalanx)
Extensor hallucis brevis	Superolateral surface of the calcaneus	Dorsum of base of proximal phalanx of the great toe
Extensor hallucis longus	Middle half of the anterior surface of the fibula and the interosseous membrane	Base of the distal phalanx of the great toe
Fibularis (peroneus) brevis	Lower one-third of the lateral surface of the fibula	Tuberosity of the base of the 5th metatarsal
Fibularis (peroneus) longus	Upper two-third of the lateral surface of the fibula	After crossing the plantar surface of the foot deep to the intrinsic muscles, it inserts on the medial cuneiform and the base of the 1st metatarsal bone
Fibularis (peroneus) tertius	Distal part of the anterior surface of the fibula	Dorsum of the shaft of the 5th metatarsal bone
Flexor digitorum longus	Middle half of the posterior surface of the tibia	Bases of the distal phalanges of digits 2-5
Flexor hallucis longus	Lower 2/3rd of the posterior surface of the fibula	Base of the distal phalanx of the great toe

Contd...

Contd...

Gastrocnemius	Femur; medial head: above the medial femoral condyle; lateral head: above the lateral femoral condyle	Dorsum of the calcaneus via the calcaneal (Achilles') tendon
Peroneus mm) (SEE fibularis mm.)		
Plantaris	Above the lateral femoral condyle (above the lateral head of gastrocnemius)	Dorsum of the calcaneus medial to the calcaneal tendon
Popliteus	Lateral condyle of the femur	Posterior surface of the tibia above soleal line
Soleus	Posterior surface of head and upper shaft of the fibula, soleal line of the tibia	Dorsum of the calcaneus via the calcaneal (Achilles') tendon
Tibialis anterior	Lateral tibial condyle and the upper lateral surface of the tibia	Medial surface of the medial cuneiform and the 1st metatarsal
Tibialis posterior	Interosseous membrane, posteromedial surface of the fibula, posterolateral surface of the tibia	Tuberosity of the navicular and medial cuneiform, metatarsals 2-4

VEINS

Vein	Tributaries	Drains into	Regions drained
Dorsal venous arch of the foot	Dorsal digital vein) and dorsal metatarsal vein	Great saphenous vein, medially, small saphenous vein laterally	Dorsum of the digits and the superficial structures of the dorsum of the foot
Greater saphenous vein	Medial end of dorsal venous arch of foot, perforating communications with deep veins, superficial epigastric vein, superficial circumflex iliac vein, superficial external pudendal vein	Femoral vein	Skin and superficial fascia of the medial side of the foot and leg; skin and superficial fascia of most of the thigh; lower abdominal wall; perineal region
Lesser saphenous vein	Lateral end of the dorsal venous arch of foot	Popliteal vein	Skin and superficial fascia of the lateral side of the foot and leg
Metatarsal, dorsal of the foot	Dorsal digital vv.	Dorsal venous arch of the foot	Dorsal aspects of the digits of the foot

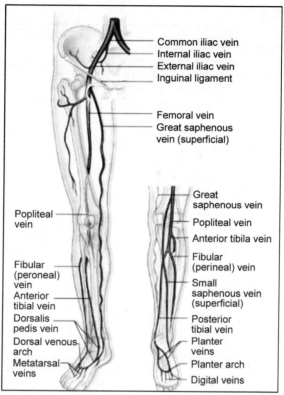

FIGURE 7.6: Diagram showing veins of lower limb

TOPOGRAPHIC ANATOMY

Structure/Space	Significance
Anterior compartment, leg	Anterior compartment of the leg contains the tibialis anterior muscle, extensor hallucis longus muscle, extensor digitorum longus muscle, fibularis tertius muscle; it also contains the anterior tibial a) and the deep fibular nerve; also known as: extensor compartment of the leg
Fascia, crural	Crural fascia is continuous with the fascia lata at the level of the knee; it is connected to the fibula by the anterior and posterior intermuscular septa; crural fascia is thickened near the ankle to form the extensor and flexor retinacula
Lateral compartment, leg	Lateral compartment of the leg contains: fibularis longus muscle, fibularis brevis muscle; superficial fibular nerve; also known as: evertor compartment of the leg
Posterior compartment, leg	Posterior compartment of the leg contains: superficially—gastrocnemius muscle, soleus muscle, plantaris muscle; deeply—popliteus muscle, tibialis posterior muscle, flexor digitorum longus muscle, flexor hallucis longus muscle; it also contains the posterior tibial a) and v) and the tibial nerve

JOINTS

Joint or ligament	Description
Ankle joint	The articulation between the distal tibia, the medial malleolus of the tibia, the lateral malleolus of the fibula and the talus
Anterior talofibular ligament	A ligament that connects the lateral malleolus of the fibula with the anterolateral surface of the talus
Anterior tibiofibular ligament	The ligament that connects the distal ends of the tibia and the fibula anteriorly
Anterior tibiotalar ligament	Part of the deltoid ligament connecting the medial malleolus of the tibia with the talus
Calcaneofibular ligament	A ligament that connects the lateral malleolus of the fibula with the calcaneus
Deltoid ligament	The ligament that connects the medial malleolus of the tibia with the talus, navicular and calcaneus
Posterior talofibular ligament	A ligament that connects the lateral malleolus of the fibula with the posterolateral surface of the talus
Posterior tibiofibular ligament	The ligament that connects the distal ends of the tibia and the fibula posteriorly
Posterior tibiotalar ligament	Part of the deltoid ligament connecting the medial malleolus of the tibia with the talus posteriorly
Tibiocalcaneal ligament	Part of the deltoid ligament connecting the medial malleolus of the tibia with the sustentaculum tali
Tibionavicular ligament	Part of the deltoid ligament connecting the medial malleolus of the tibia with the navicular

ARTERIES OF THE LOWER LIMB

Artery	Source	Supply to
Anterior tibial	Popliteal artery	Anterior leg; dorsum of foot and deep foot
Aorta, abdominal	The continuation of the descending thoracic aorta	Abdominal wall; gastrointestinal tract; body below the level of the respiratory diaphragm
Arch, plantar arterial	Lateral plantar artery	Deep foot; its plantar metatarsal brs) and their brs) supply the toes, including the dorsum of the distal phalangeal segment
Circumflex femoral, lateral	Deep femoral artery	Lateral thigh and hip
Circumflex femoral, medial	Deep femoral artery	Medial thigh and hip
Circumflex fibular	Anterior tibial	Proximal portion of lateral leg
Circumflex iliac, superficial	Femoral artery	Superficial fascia of lower abdomen and thigh
Deep external pudendal	Femoral artery	Origins of pectineus m., adductor longus m.; scrotum/labium majus
Deep femoral	Femoral artery	Hip joint, proximal thigh, posterior thigh

Contd...

Contd...

Descending genicular	Femoral artery	Skin and superficial structures of the medial aspect of the knee and upper leg
Digital, proper plantar	Plantar metatarsal artery, from the plantar arterial arch	Plantar aspect of each digit
Dorsal metatarsal	Dorsalis pedis (1st), arcuate (2nd-4th)	Dorsum of digits, excluding the distal phalangeal segment
Dorsalis pedis	Anterior tibial artery	Dorsal aspect of the foot;
External iliac	Common iliac artery	Lower limb
External pudendal, deep	Femoral artery	Origins of pectineus m., adductor longus m.; scrotum/labium majus
External pudendal, superficial	Femoral artery	Skin and superficial fascia of the upper medial thigh, skin of the pubic region
Femoral	External iliac artery	Thigh, leg and foot
Femoral, deep	Femoral artery	Hip joint, proximal thigh, posterior thigh
Femoral, lateral circumflex	Deep femoral artery	Lateral thigh and hip
Femoral, medial circumflex	Deep femoral artery	Medial thigh and hip
Fibular	Posterior tibial artery	Muscles and fascia of the lateral leg ankle
Genicular, descending	Femoral artery	Skin and superficial structures of the medial aspect of the knee and upper leg

Contd...

Contd...

Gluteal, inferior	Internal iliac artery, anterior division		Gluteus maximus m., hip joint
Gluteal, superior	Internal iliac, posterior division		Gluteus maximus m., gluteus medius m., gluteus minimus m., hip joint
Iliac, common	Abdominal aorta		Pelvis, lower limb
Iliac, external	Common iliac artery	Inferior epigastric artery, deep circumflex iliac artery, femoral artery	Lower limb
Iliolumbar	Internal iliac artery, posterior division	Iliac br., lumbar br.	Iliacus m., psoas major m., quadratus lumborum m.
Inferior epigastric	External iliac artery	Cremasteric artery	Lower rectus abdominis m., pyramidalis m., lower abdominal wall
Inferior gluteal	Internal iliac artery, anterior division	Unnamed muscular branches	Gluteus maximus m., hip joint
Inferior lateral genicular	Popliteal artery	No named branches	Lateral aspect of the knee
Inferior medial genicular	Popliteal artery	No named branches	Medial aspect of the knee

Contd...

Contd...

Metatarsal, dorsal	Dorsalis pedis (1st), arcuate (2nd-4th)	Dorsal digital aa) (2)	Dorsum of digits, excluding the distal phalangeal segment
Metatarsal, plantar	Plantar arterial arch	Perforating br., plantar digital aa) (2)	Interosseous mm., deep portions of the foot; digits including the dorsum of the distal phalangeal segment
Obturator	Internal iliac artery, anterior division		Medial thigh and hip
Plantar arterial arch	Lateral plantar artery		Deep foot; its plantar metatarsal brs) and their brs) supply the toes, including the dorsum of the distal phalangeal segment
Plantar, deep	Dorsalis pedis		Deep foot; its plantar metatarsal brs) and their brs) supply the toes, including the dorsum of the distal phalangeal segment
Plantar, lateral	Posterior tibial artery		Deep foot; the plantar arterial arch and its brs) supply the toes, including the distal phalangeal segment dorsally
Plantar, medial	Posterior tibial artery		Medial side of the sole of the foot
Popliteal	Femoral artery		Knee, leg and foot

Contd...

Contd...

Posterior tibial	Popliteal artery	Posterior and lateral leg, plantar aspect of the foot
Pudendal, superficial external	Femoral artery	Skin and superficial fascia of the upper medial thigh, skin of the pubic region

Contd...

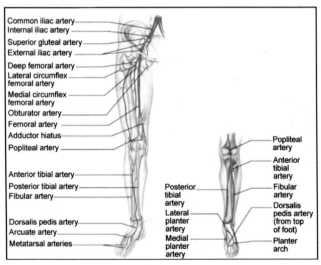

FIGURE 7.7: Arteries of lower limb

Contd...

Superficial epigastric	Femoral artery	Superficial fascia and skin of the lower abdominal wall
Superficial external pudendal	Femoral artery	Skin and superficial fascia of the upper medial thigh, skin of the pubic region
Tarsal, lateral	Dorsalis pedis artery	Tarsal bones and joints of the lateral foot
Tarsal, medial	Dorsalis pedis artery	Tarsal bones and joints of the medial side of the foot
Tibial, anterior	Popliteal artery	Anterior leg; dorsum of foot and deep foot
Tibial, posterior	Popliteal artery	Posterior and lateral leg, plantar aspect of the foot

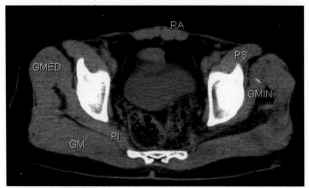

FIGURE 7.8: Axial sections at the level of acetabular roof. RA—Rectus abdominus, PS—Psoa S, GMED—Gluteus medius, GM—Gluteus maximus, PI—Piriformis, GMIN—Gluteus minimus

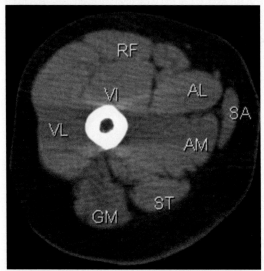

FIGURE 7.9: Axial CT at the level of proximal thigh. SA—Sartorius, RF—Rectus femoris, AL—Adductor longus, AM—Adductor magnus, ST—Semitendinosus, Gm—Gluteus maximus, VL—Vastus lateralls, VI—Vastus intermedius

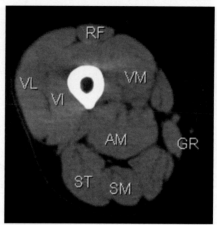

FIGURE 7.10: Axial CT at the level of distal thigh. RF—Rectus femoris, VM—Vastus medialis, GR—Gracilis, AM—Adductor magnus, VL—Vastus lateralis, VI—Vastus intermedius, ST—Semitendinosis, SM—Semimembranosis

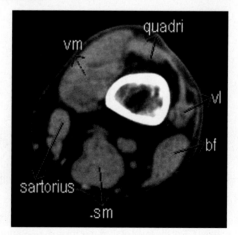

FIGURE 7.11: Axial CT at the suprapatellar level. VM—Vastus Medialis, Qudri—audriceps, VI—Vastus Lateralis, BF—Biceps Femoris, SM—Semimembranosus

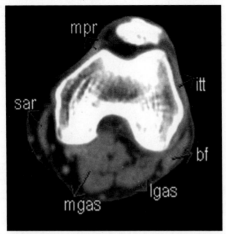

FIGURE 7.12: Axial CT at the patellar level. Sar—Sartorius, itt—iliotitrial tract, bf—Biceps femoris, mgas—Medial head of gastrocnemius, lgas—Lateral head of gastronemius, MPR—Medial patellar retinaculum

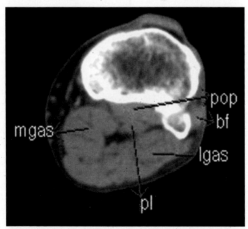

FIGURE 7.13: Axial CT at the level of tibial plateu: Pop—Popletius, bf—Biceps femoris, lgas—Lateral head of gastrocnemius, mgas—Medial head of gastrocnemius, pl—Peroneus longus

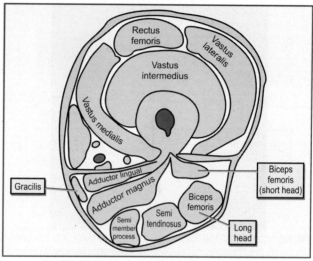

FIGURE 7.14: Cross-section at the mid thigh level

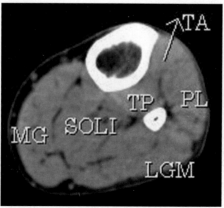

FIGURE 7.15: Axial CT at mid leg level. TA—Tibialis anterior, TP—Titrialis posterior, PL—Peroneus longus, SOLI—Soleus, MG—Medial gastrocnemius, LGM—Lateral gastrocnemius

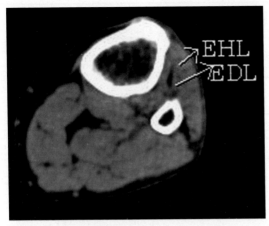

FIGURE 7.16: Axial CT at lower leg level. EHL—Extensor hallucis longus, EDL—Extensor digitorum longus

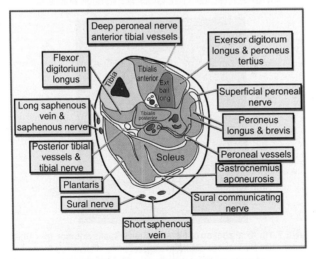

FIGURE 7.17: Axial (cross) section lower leg

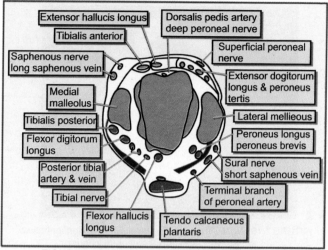

FIGURE 7.18: Axial (cross) section through right ankle

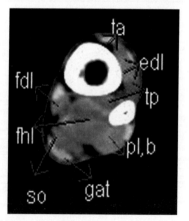

FIGURE 7.19: Axial section of distal leg. ta—Tibialis anterior, tp—Tibialis posterior, EDL—Extensor digitrium longus, pl, b—Peroneus longus and brevius, fdl—Flexor digitorum longus, fhl—Flexor hallucis longus, SO—Soleus, gat—Medial gastrocnemius

BONES OF FOOT

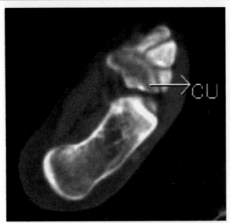

FIGURE 7.20: Cu—Cuneiform

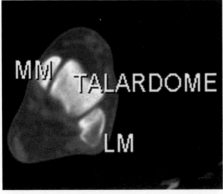

FIGURE 7.21: MM—Medial Malleolus, LM—Lateral Malleolus

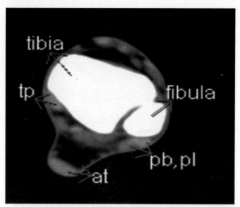

FIGURE 7.22: at—Achillestendon

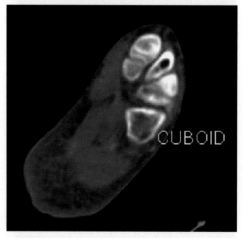

FIGURE 7.23: Cuboid

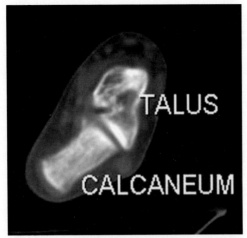

FIGURE 7.24: Calcaneum

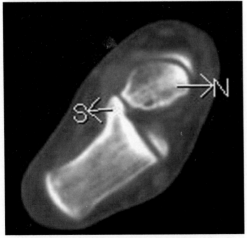

FIGURE 7.25: Bones of foot. N—Naviceler,
S—Sustentaculumtali, Talus

Chapter 8

Upper Limb

OSTEOLOGY OF THE ARM AND ELBOW REGION

Bone	Structure	Description
Humerus		The humerus articulates proximally with the scapula at the glenoid fossa; it articulates distally with the radius and ulna at the elbow joint
	Head	It articulates with the glenoid cavity of the scapula to form the shoulder joint
	Anatomical neck	It is located at the circumference of the smooth articular surface of the head
	Surgical neck	It is located inferior to the greater and lesser tubercles; it is a site of frequent fracture; fractures of the surgical neck of the humerus endanger the axillary nerve and the posterior circumflex humeral vessels
	Greater tubercle	It is the attachment site of the supraspinatus, infraspinatus and teres minor mm. which are three members of the rotator cuff group
	Lesser tubercle	It is the insertion site of the subscapularis muscle, a member of the rotator cuff group
	Crest of the greater tubercle	It forms the lateral lip of the intertubercular groove; it is the attachment site for the transverse humeral ligament and the pectoralis major muscle.
	Crest of the lesser tubercle	It forms the medial lip of the intertubercular groove; it is the attachment site for the transverse humeral ligament and the teres major muscle.
	Intertubercular groove	It is occupied by the tendon of the long head of the biceps brachii muscle; the transverse humeral ligament spans the intertubercular groove and holds the tendon of the long head of the biceps in

Contd...

Contd...

	place; it is the attachment site for the tendon of the pectoralis major (lateral lip), teres major (medial lip), and latissimus dorsi (floor)
Deltoid tuberosity	It is the insertion site of the deltoid m.
Radial groove	It is a depression for the radial n. and the deep brachial vessels; fracture of the humerus at mid-shaft can injure the radial nerve and deep brachial vessels because they are in contact with bone at this location
Lateral epicondyle	It is the site of attachment of the common extensor tendon which is the origin of several forearm extensor muscles (extensor carpi radialis brevis m., extensor digitorum m., extensor digiti minimi m. and extensor carpi ulnaris m.); inflammation of the attachment of the common extensor tendon is called lateral epicondylitis which is also known as "tennis elbow"
Medial epicondyle	It is the attachment site of the common flexor tendon which is the origin for the superficial group of forearm flexor muscles (pronator teres m., flexor carpi radialis m., palmaris longus m., flexor carpi ulnaris m. and flexor digitorum superficialis m.); inflammation of the attachment of the common flexor tendon is called medial epicondylitis; the ulnar nerve is in contact with bone as it courses posterior to the medial epicondyle where it is susceptible to injury from blunt trauma or fracture
Medial supra-condylar ridge	The pronator teres m. takes origin from the common flexor tendon near the most inferior part of the medial supracondylar ridge

Contd...

Contd...

	Lateral supra-condylar ridge	It is the site of origin of the brachio-radialis m. and the extensor carpi radialis longus m.
	Coronoid fossa	It accommodates the coronoid process of ulna when the elbow is flexed
	Radial fossa	It accommodates the head of the radius when the elbow is flexed
	Olecranon fossa	It accommodates the olecranon process of the ulna when the elbow is extended
	Capitulum	It articulates with the head of the radius; capitulum means "little head"
	Trochlea	It articulates with the trochlear notch of the ulna; the shape of the trochlea and the trochlear notch limits side-to-side movement and guarantees a hinge action; trochlea means "pulley"
Ulna		The ulna articulates proximally with the trochlea of the humerus and the head of the radius; it articulates distally with the ulnar notch of the radius
	Olecranon	It is the insertion site of the tendon of the triceps brachii m.; when the elbow is extended, the olecranon of the ulna engages the olecranon fossa of the humerus
	Trochlear notch	It is located between the olecranon and the coronoid process; it articulates with the trochlea of the humerus; a ridge within the trochlear notch fits into the groove in the trochlea of the humerus which limits side-to-side movement and guarantees a hinge action
	Coronoid process	It is the insertion site of the brachialis m.
	Radial notch	It accommodates the head of the radius; the ends of the annular ligament attach to the anterior and posterior edges of the radial notch of the ulna to encircle the head of the radius

Contd...

Contd...

	Body	It is also called the shaft or diaphysis; the interosseous membrane attaches to the entire length of the interosseous border of the body of the ulna
	Head	It is small and rounded for articulation with the radius
	Styloid process	It is the site of attachment of the articular disk of the distal radioulnar joint
Radius		The radius pivots on its long axis and crosses the ulna during pronation
	Head	It has a smooth, rounded surface for articulation with the ulna; the head of the radius is encircled by the annular ligament (4/5 of a circle) and the radial notch of the ulna (1/5 of a circle)
	Neck	The annular ligament of the radius surrounds the head of the radius, not the neck of the radius
	Radial tuberosity	It is the insertion site of the tendon of the biceps brachii m.
	Body	It is also known as the shaft or diaphysis; the interosseous membrane attaches to the entire length of the body of the radius along its interosseous border; a fracture of the distal end of the body of the radius with a dorsal displacement of the distal fragment is quite common and is called a Colles' fracture
	Ulnar notch	It articulates with the head of the ulna
	Styloid process	The radial styloid process projects lateral to the proximal row of carpal bones

MUSCLES OF THE ARM

Muscle	Origin	Insertion
Anconeus	Lateral epicondyle of the humerus	Lateral side of the olecranon and the upper one-fourth of the ulna
Biceps brachii	Short head: tip of the coracoid process of the scapula; long head: supraglenoid tubercle of the scapula	Tuberosity of the radius
Brachialis	Anterior surface of the lower one-half of the humerus and the associated intermuscular septa	Coronoid process of the ulna
Coracobrachialis	Coracoid process of the scapula	Medial side of the humerus at mid-shaft
Triceps brachii	Long head: infraglenoid tubercle of the scapula; lateral head: posterolateral humerus and lateral intermuscular septum; medial head: posteromedial surface of the inferior 1/2 of the humerus	Olecranon process of the ulna

ARTERIES OF THE ARM AND ELBOW REGION

Artery	Source	Branches	Supply to
Anterior circumflex humeral	Axillary artery, 3rd part	Unnamed muscular branches	Deltoid muscle; arm muscles near the surgical neck of the humerus
Brachial	Axillary artery (brachial artery is the continuation of the axillary artery distal to the teres major muscle)	Deep brachial artery, superior ulnar collateral artery, nutrient artery, inferior ulnar collateral artery; terminal branches are the radial artery and the ulnar artery	Arm, forearm and hand
Brachial, deep	Brachial artery	Ascending branch.; terminal branches are the middle collateral artery and radial collateral artery	Muscles and tissues of the posterior compartment of the arm
Collateral, inferior ulnar	Brachial artery	Unnamed muscular branches	Lower medial arm
Collateral, middle	Deep brachial artery	Unnamed muscular branches	Medial head of triceps, anconeus
Collateral, radial	Deep brachial artery	Unnamed muscular branches	Lower lateral arm
Collateral, superior ulnar	Brachial artery	Unnamed muscular branches	Medial arm muscles
Posterior circumflex humeral	Axillary artery, 3rd part	Unnamed muscular branches	Deltoid; arm muscles near the surgical neck of the humerus

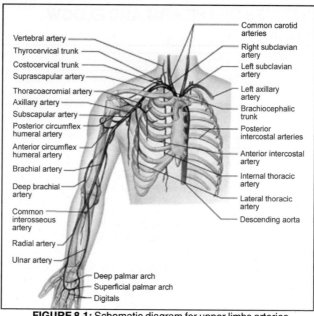

FIGURE 8.1: Schematic diagram for upper limbs arteries

VEINS OF THE ELBOW REGION

Vein	Tributaries	Drains into	Regions drained
Basilic vein	Medial end of the dorsal venous arch of the hand; superficial veins of the forearm; median cubital vein	It unites with the brachial vein(s) to form the axillary vein	Superficial parts of the medial side of the hand and medial side of the forearm
Cephalic vein	Lateral side of the dorsal venous arch of the hand; superficial veins of the forearm	Axillary vein	
Median cubital vein	Cephalic	Basilic	

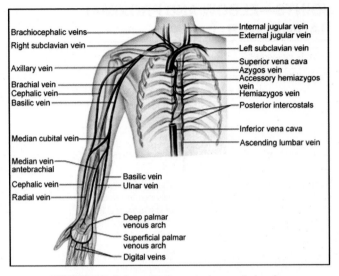

FIGURE 8.2: Schematic diagram of upper limb veins

JOINTS—ELBOW AND PROXIMAL RADIOULNAR

Joint or ligament	Description
Elbow joint	The joint between the distal humerus and the proximal radius and ulna
Radioulnar joint, distal	The articulation between the head of the ulna and the ulnar notch of the radius
Radioulnar joint, intermediate	The articulation formed by the interosseous membrane
Radioulnar joint, proximal	The proximal articulation between the radius and ulna that is contained within the capsule of the elbow joint

ELBOW JOINT (ANTEROPOSTERIOR)

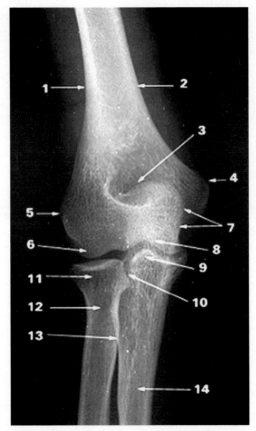

FIGURE 8.3: Elbow Joint (Anteroposterior). (1) Lateral supracondylar ridge, (2) Medial supracondylar ridge, (3) Olecranon fossa, (4) Medial epicondyle, (5) Lateral epicondyle, (6) Capitulum, (7) Olecranon, (8) Trochlea, (9) Coronoid process of ulna, (10) Proximal radioulnar joint, (11) Head of radius, (12) Neck of radius, (13) Tuberosity of radius, (14) Ulna

ELBOW JOINT (LATERAL)

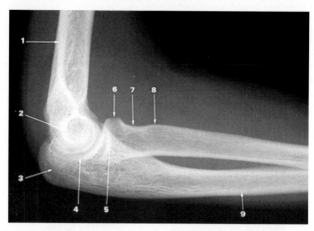

FIGURE 8.4: Elbow joing (lateral). (1) Supracondylar ridge, (2) Trochlea, (3) Olecranon, (4) Trochlear notch, (5) Coronoid process of ulna, (6) Head of radius, (7) Neck of radius, (8) Tuberosity of radius, (9) Ulna

FOREARM (ANTEROPOSTERIOR)

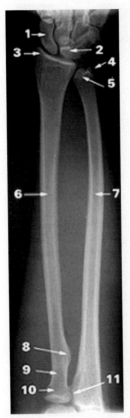

FIGURE 8.5: Forearm (Anteroposterior. (1) Scaphoid, (2) Lunate, (3) Styloid process of radius, (4) Styloid process of ulna, (5) Head of ulna, (6) Radius, (7) Ulna, (8) Tuberosity of radius, (9) Neck of radius, (10) Head of radius, (11) Proximal radioulnar joint

FOREARM (LATERAL)

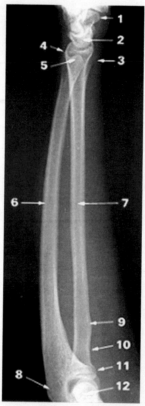

FIGURE 8.6: Forearm (lateral). (1) Scaphoid, (2) Lunate, (3) Distal end of radius, (4) Styloid process of ulna, (5) Head of ulna, (6) Ulna, (7) Radius, (8) Olecranon, (9) Tuberosity of radius, (10) Neck of radius, (11) Head of radius, (12) Trochlea

SHOULDER JOINT (ANTEROPOSTERIOR)

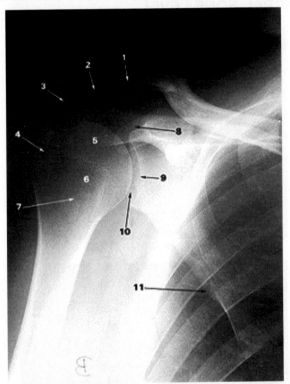

FIGURE 8.7: Shoulder joint (Anteroposterior) (1) Clavicle, (2) Acromioclavicular joint, (3) Acromion, (4) Greater tubercle of humerus, (5) Head of humerus, (6) Lesser tubercle of humerus, (7) Surgical neck of humerus, (8) Coracoid process, (9) Glenoid fossa, (10) Shoulder joint, (11) Lateral border of scapula

AXIAL SECTIONS THROUGH THE WRIST— CARPAL BONE LEVEL

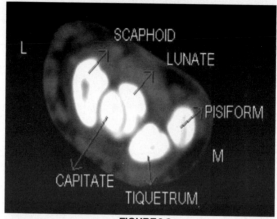

FIGURE 8.8

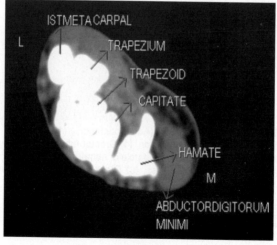

FIGURE 8.9

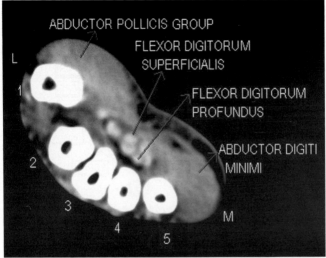

FIGURE 8.10: Axial sections at metacarpal level

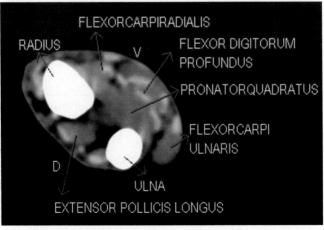

FIGURE 8.11: Axial section at the level of radius and ulna

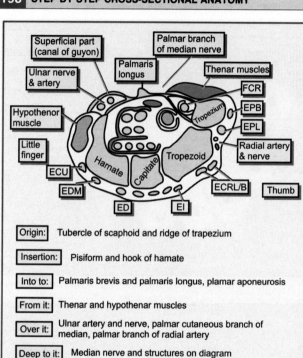

Origin:	Tubercle of scaphoid and ridge of trapezium
Insertion:	Pisiform and hook of hamate
Into to:	Palmaris brevis and palmaris longus, plamar aponeurosis
From it:	Thenar and hypothenar muscles
Over it:	Ulnar artery and nerve, palmar cutaneous branch of median, palmar branch of radial artery
Deep to it:	Median nerve and structures on diagram
Note:	Synovial sheaths open laterally to allow for small vessels to tendons

FIGURE 8.12: Schematic diagram at the level of wrist

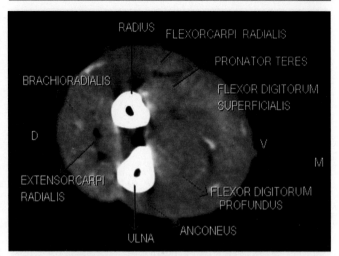

FIGURE 8.13: Axial sections of proximal forearm

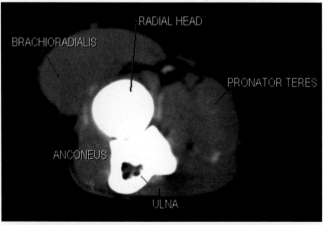

FIGURE 8.14: Axial sections at the level of radial head

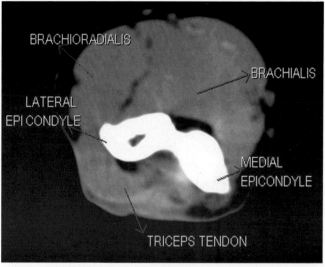

FIGURE 8.15: Axial sections through distal humerus

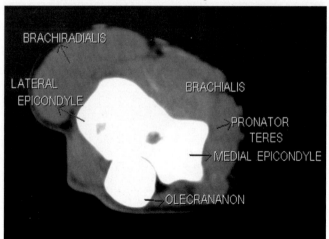

FIGURE 8.16: Axial CT at the level of olecranon

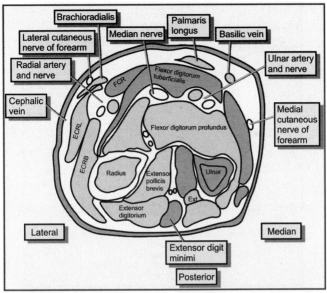

FIGURE 8.17: Axial schematic at the level of distal forearm

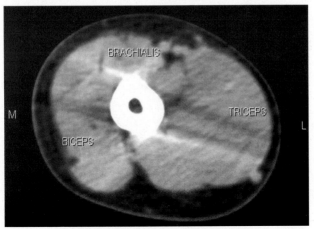

FIGURE 8.18: Axial section through midarm

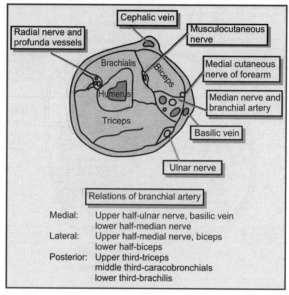

FIGURE 8.19: Schematic diagram at the level of midarm

AXIAL SECTIONS THROUGH THE SHOULDER JOINTS

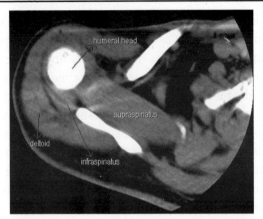

FIGURE 8.20: Axial section at the level of humeral head

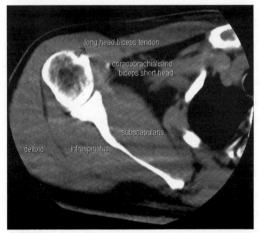

FIGURE 8.21: Axial section at the level of shoulder joint

MUSCLES AROUND THE SHOULDER JOINT

Subscapularis Muscle

This is one of the muscles of the rotator cuff, which is a group of four muscles also including the supraspinatus, infraspinatus, and teres minor. These four muscles are responsible for providing stability for the shoulder joint by holding the head of the humerus in the glenoid cavity of the scapula. The subscapularis sits anterior to the scapula and posterior to the serratus anterior muscle. The origin of this muscle is located at the subscapular fossa of the scapula. The muscle inserts in the lesser tubercle of the humerus. The action of the muscle is medial rotation and adduction of the arm. The muscles is enervated by the lower subscapular nerve (C5-C7).

Infraspinatus Muscle

This muscle is also one of the members of the rotator cuff group. It originates from the dorsal aspect of the scapula and inserts into the greater tubercle of the humerus. It also sits inferior to the spine of the scapula. Its action is to laterally rotate the arm and also help stabilize the shoulder joint. It is enervated by the subscapular nerve.

Supraspinatus Muscle

It originates in the supraspinatus fossa of the scapula, which is located above the spine of the scapula. The muscle inserts into the superior aspect of the greater tubercle of the humerus. It is innervated by the subscapular nerve. The actions of the muscle include helping the deltoid muscles to abduct the arm. As with other rotator cuff muscles, it helps stabilize the shoulder joint.

Teres Minor Muscle

It originates from the superior part of the lateral border of the scapula and inserts in the greater tubercle of the humerus. Like the teres major, the teres minor is located also below the spine of the scapula. It serves to adduct and medially rotate the arm. It is enervated by the axillary nerve. It sits superior to the teres major muscle.

Chapter 9

Skull Base

INTRODUCTION

The skull base is formed of the membranous bones and cartilage perforated by nerves, arteries and veins. Skull base consists of anterior, middle and posterior compartments.

ANTERIOR CRANIAL FOSSA

- Boundaries
- Contents
  - Orbital plate of frontal bone
  - Cribriform plate of the ethmoid bone
  - Crista galli of the ethmoid bone
  - Lesser wing of the sphenoid bone
  - Foramen cecum

MIDDLE CRANIAL FOSSA

- Boundaries
- Contents
  - Body of the sphenoid bone
  - Sella turcica
    - Anterior clinoid processes
    - Dorsum sellae
    - Posterior clinoid processes
  - Greater wing of sphenoid
  - Squamous part of the temporal bone
  - Carotid canal and groove
  - Petrous part of the temporal bone
  - Orbital fissures
    - Superior
    - Inferior

- Foramina
  - Rotundum
  - Ovale
  - Spinosum
- Optic canal
- Hiatus of the facial canal

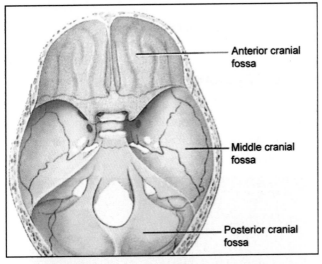

FIGURE 9.1: Schematic diagram showing skull base

POSTERIOR CRANIAL FOSSA

- Boundaries
- Contents
  - Occipital bone
  - Petrous part of the temporal bone
  - Dorsum sellae
  - Clivus
  - Jugular foramen

- Hypoglossal canal
- Internal auditory meatus
- Foramen magnum
- Condyloid canal
- Grooves for:
  - Sigmoid sinus
  - Transverse sinus
  - Superior sagittal sinus
  - Occipital sinus

SKULL BASE FORAMINA

On the inner aspect of middle cranial fossa 3 foramina are oriented along an oblique line in the greater sphenoidal wing from anteromedial behind the superior orbital fissure to the posterolateral.

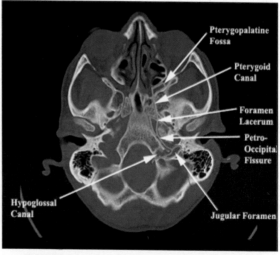

FIGURE 9.2: Axial CT showing skull base foramina

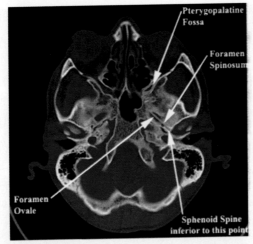

FIGURE 9.3: Axial CT showing skull base foramina

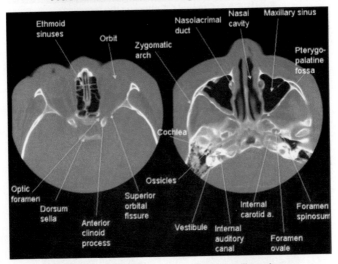

FIGURE 9.4:: Axial CT at the level of maxillary sinus

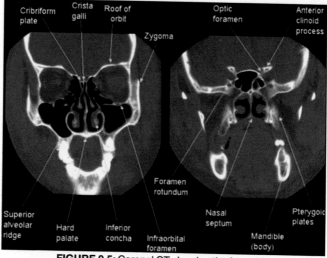

FIGURE 9.5: Coronal CT showing the foramina

SCHEMATIC OF THE CRANIAL NERVES

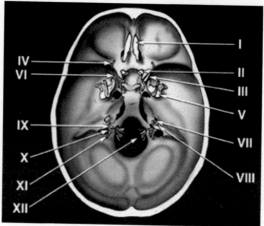

FIGURE 9.6: Schematic diagram showing cranial nerve foramina

CORONAL CECT AT THE LEVEL OF CAVERNOUS SINUS (ARROW)

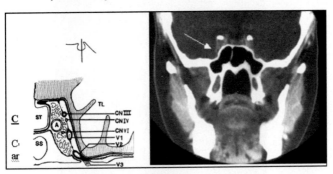

FIGURE 9.7

CORONAL AND AXIAL CT SECTIONS SHOWING THE FORAMEN OVALE

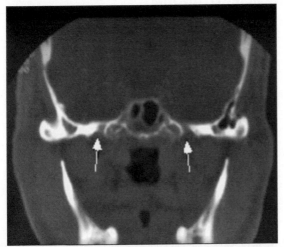

FIGURE 9.8: *Contents* – fifth nerve third division, lesser petrosal nerve, accessory meningeal artery, emissary veins.

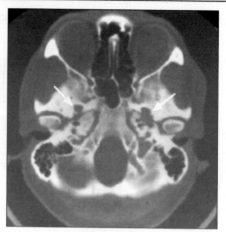

FIGURE 9.9

CORONAL SECTIONS AT THE LEVEL OF FORAMEN ROTUNDUM

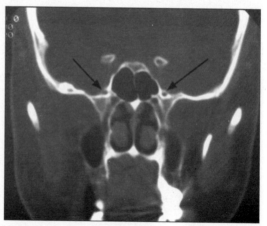

FIGURE 9.10: *Contents*—fifth nerve second division, emissary veins, artery of foramen of rotundum.

AXIAL SECTIONS OF THE INFRAORBITAL CANAL

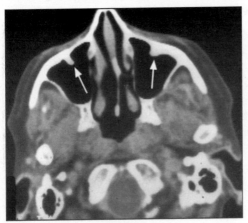

FIGURE 9.11

AXIAL SECTION AT THE LEVEL OF THE PTERYGO-PALATINE FOSSA

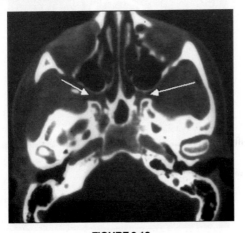

FIGURE 9.12

Coronal sections showing 1) superior orbital fissure 2) inferior orbital fissure

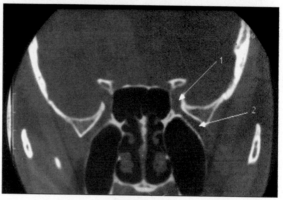

FIGURE 9.13

AXIAL SECTIONS SHOWING THE OPTIC CANAL

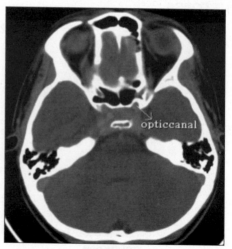

FIGURE 9.14

AXIAL SECTIONS SHOWING THE SKULL BASE ARTICULATION

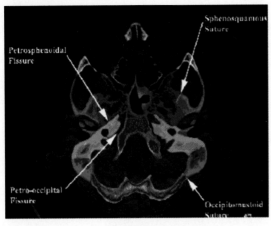

FIGURE 9.15

RED—TEMPORAL   VIOLET–OCCIPITAL
GREEN–SPHENOID   ORANGE–PETROUS BONE

Chapter 10

Cervical Spine

INTRODUCTION

The first and second cervical vertebrae are functionally and morphologically distinct, atlas is an osseous ring with paired articulating facets for matching articular surfaces of the occipital bone c2 has an elongated body that continues superiorly as dens. dens articulates anteriorly with anterior arch of c1, c3 – c7 vertebrae have moderate wedge shape in mid saggital sections c5 body is smallest.

The lateral margins of the superior end plate of c3 to c7 form a short bony wall that extend anteroposteriorly and curves around the posterolateral corner of each endplate (uncinate process). There is an articulating facet on the lateral side of the inferior end plates usually c2-c6, that articulate with the uncinate process of the next caudad cervical body to form the uncovertebral joint of Luschka. The transverse process of each cervical vertebrae contains the foramen transversorium anterolaterally through which the vertebral artery passes through.

The cervical facetal joints are oriented in their anterior portions at a 10-20 degree tilt to the vertical in the cervical spine the facetal joints are situated on the posterior aspect of each neural foraminae. The cervical neural foramina are located 45 degrees to the sagittal plane.

DORSAL SPINE

The thoracic vertebral bodies are usually somewhat flatter anteroposteriorly than the cervical bodies the vertebrae gradually increase in width and height from the upper to the lower thoracic level, on mid sagittal cross sections they

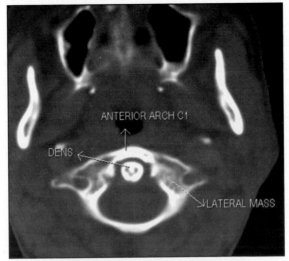

FIGURE 10.1: Axial section at the level of c1

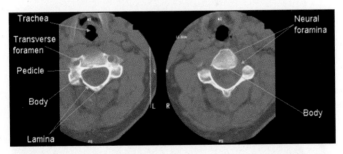

FIGURE 10.2: Axial sections at the level of body and neural foramina

are moderately wedge shaped. The basivertebral vein is fairly prominent in the thoracic region.

An important feature of the dorsal vertebrae is the costocentral articulation between each rib and the body,

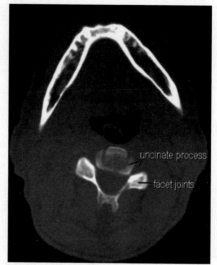

FIGURE 10.3: Axial sections at inferior end plate

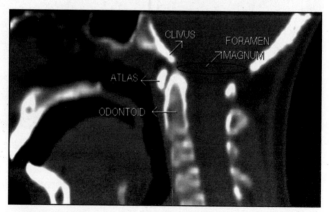

FIGURE 10.4: Coronal reformation of craniovertebral junction

costotransverse articulation between the rib and the transverse process.

Neural foramina extend from the spinal canal at an angle of 90 degress to the sagittal.

Facetal joints have an oblique axial orientation in the upper thoracic region and gradually becomes oblique coronal orientation.

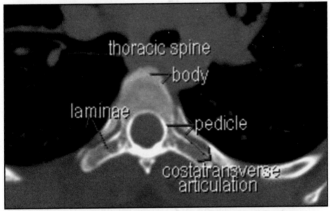

FIGURE 10.5: Axial sections of dorsal spine level of body

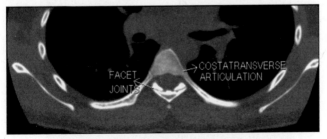

FIGURE 10.6: Axial sections at the level of facetal joint

LUMBAR SPINE

Lumbar vertebral bodies increase in size from L1-L4. The posterior surfaces of L1-L3 vertebrae have a distinct axial concavity in the middle. The posterior sufaces of l4 and l5 may be flat or convex, neural foraminae are oriented in the coronal plane, facetal joints are in an oblique plane. the anterolateral portion of the spinal canal is called the lateral recess.

AXIAL SECTONS AT THE LEVEL OF BODY

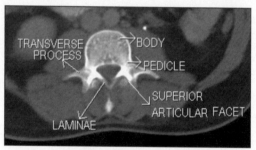

FIGURE 10.7: Lumbar vertebrae

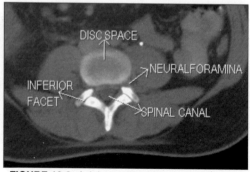

FIGURE 10.8: Axial sectons at the level of disc space

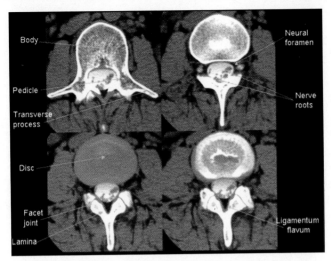

FIGURE 10.9: Axial sections of CT myelogram at the L1 level
showing the nerve roots of cauda equina

SACRUM

The sacrum is formed by the fusion of five sacral vertebrae.
The spinal canal continues as the central canal of sacrum.
The sacral neural foramina are situated lateral to the sacral
canal.

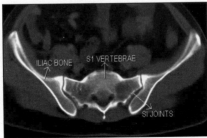

FIGURE 10.10: Axial sections at the level of s1 vertebrae

BASICS

Chapter 11

Orbits

Orbital volume and dimensions: = 30 cc, 35 (Height) × 45 (Width) × 45 mm(medial wall depth), globe 25 × 25 mm

Bones: (F)rontal, (M)axillary, (Z)ygomatic, (L)acrimal, (E)thmoid, (P)alatine, (S)phenoid

ROOF

- Bones
  - Frontal
  - Lesser wing of sphenoid
- Contents
  - Lacrimal gland fossa
  - Trochlea 4 mm posterior to margin for superior oblique tendon
- Supraorbital notch/foramen
- Clinical Correlations
  - Subperisteal abscess

MEDIAL WALL

- Bones
  - Maxillary
  - Lacrimal
  - Ethmoid-thinnest
  - Sphenoid
- Contents
  - Lacrimal sac fossa
  - Cribiform plate is medial to anterior orbit at the level of fronto-ethmoidal suture

FLOOR

- Bones
  - Maxillary- second thinnest, thins posteriorly
    - Zygoma
    - Palatine
- Contents
  - Infraorbital foramen
  - Inferior oblique origin
  - Slopes 20 degrees down
  - Suspensory ligament of eyeball

LATERAL WALL

- Bones
  - Zygomatic bone
  - Greater wing of sphenoid
- Contents
  - Lateral orbital tubercle is 11 mm below F-Z suture,
  - Serves as attachment of check ligament of lateral rectus

HOLES AND FISSURES

- Fissures
  - Superior orbital fissure (SOF):
    - 22 mm long
    - Separates greater wing of sphenoid from lesser wing of sphenoid
    - Transmits third, fourth, sixth and V1 and sympathetic fibers

- lateral rectus origin separates into superior and inferior divisions
  - Superior division transmits lacrimal, frontal and trochlear nerves
  - Inferior division transmits superior and inferior divisions of CN III, nasociliary branch of CN V, CN IV, superior ophthalmic vein, and sympathetic nerve plexus
- Venous system: superior ophthalmic vein
  - Inferior orbital fissure (IOF)
  - Located between lateral orbital wall and the orbital floor
  - Transmits V_2 (maxillary), pterygoid nerves nerve arising from pterygopalatine ganglion
  - Infraorbital nerve (a branch of V_2) enters the infraobital groove and infraorbital canal for sensation to lower eyelid, cheek, upper lid, upper teeth
  - Venous system inferior ophthalmic vein

HOLES/NOTCHES/CANALS

- Nasolacrimal canal
  - Lacrimal sac fossa to the inferior meatus
  - Separates greater wing of sphenoid from lesser wing of sphenoid
  - Transmits third, fourth, sixth and V1 and symphathetic fibers
  - Lateral rectus origin separates into superior and inferior divisions

- Superior division transmits lacrimal, frontal and trochlear nerves
- Inferior division transmits superior and inferior divisions of CN III, nasociliary branch of CN V, CN IV, superior ophthalmic vein, and sympathetic nerve plexus
- Venous system: superior ophthalmic vein
- Supraorbital foramen/notch
  - Transmits blood vessels
  - Supraorbital nerve
  - Anterior/posterior ethmoidal foramen: transmits ethmoidal blood vessels and nerve
  - Zygomatic foramen: transmits zygomaticofrontal and zygomaticotemporal nerves, zygomatic artery
  - Nasolacrimal duct (NLD): exits into inferior meatus
  - Infraorbital canal: transmits infraorbital nerve (V_2)
  - Ethmoidal foramina
    - Anterior ethmoidal artery
    - Posterior ethmoidal artery
    - Allows infections and neoplasms to enter to orbit from the sinuses
  - Optic canal
    - 8-10 mm long
    - Located within the less wing of sphenoid
    - Separated from SOF by OPTIC STRUT

- Transmits ophthalmic nerve, ophthalmic artery, sympathetic nerves
- Optic foramen is 6.5 mm wide: it may be enlarged in the presence of optic nerve glioma; 1 mm of asymmetry between right and left is abnormal

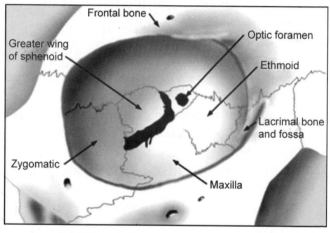

FIGURE 11.1: Diagram showing bones of orbit

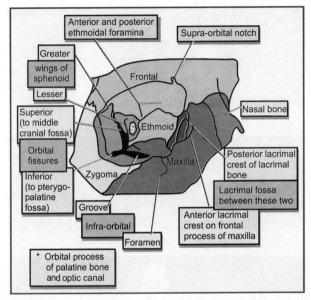

FIGURE 11.2

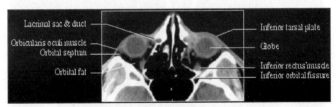

FIGURE 11.3: Axial CT of orbit

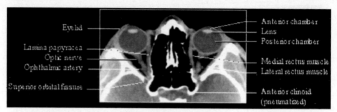

FIGURE 11.4

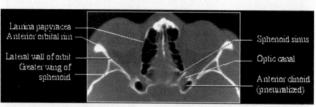

FIGURE 11.5: Axial sections of orbit

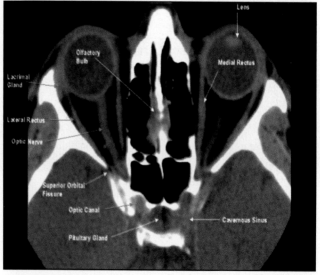

FIGURE 11.6: Axial sections at the level of superior orbital fissure

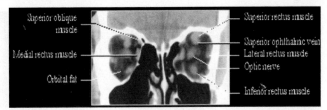

FIGURE 11.7

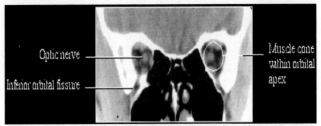

FIGURE 11.8

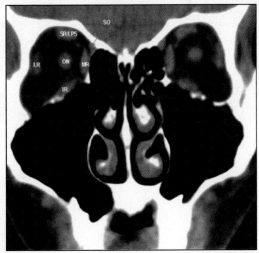

FIGURES 11.8 and 11.9: Coronal sections of orbit showing
intraocular muscles

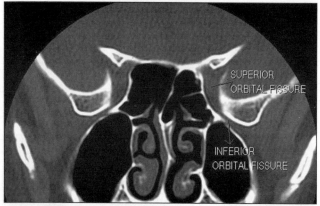

FIGURE 11.10: Coronal CT showing orbital fissures

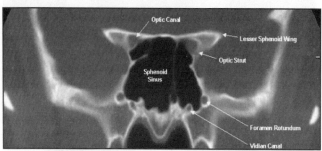

FIGURE 11.11: Coronal CT showing optic canal

Chapter 12

Cardiac CT Anatomy

The first coronary artery seen (starting superiorly from its origin) is the LMA. The LMA arises from the left sinus of Valsalva and courses to the left posterior to the main pulmonary artery. The LMA bifurcates into the LAD and the LCX. The LAD runs anteriorly in the anterior interventricular groove. The LAD gives off septal and diagonal branches. The LCX runs to the left and inferiorly in the posterior atrioventricular groove The LCX gives off marginal branches, which supply the left ventricle.

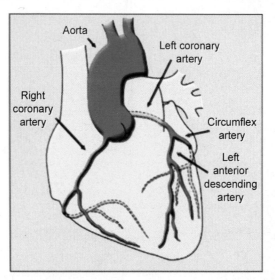

FIGURE 12.1: Diagram showing coronary arteries

The RCA originates more caudally from the aorta than the LMA. The RCA arises from the right sinus of Valsalva . The RCA runs anteriorly and to the right, and then courses inferiorly. The RCA runs in the anterior atrioventricular groove. The RCA and LCX can be followed inferiorly toward the apex of the heart.

The PDA usually arises from the RCA. Coronary artery dominance is defined by which coronary artery gives rise to the PDA. The RCA is dominant in 70% of people with the RCA giving rise to the PDA.

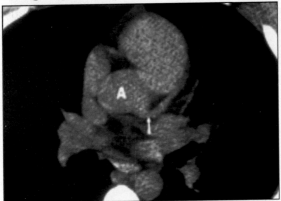

FIGURE 12.2: Left main coronary artery—plain CT scan

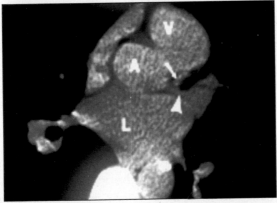

FIGURE 12.3: Bifurcation of the LMA into the LAD (arrow) and the LCX (arrowhead)—plain CT scan

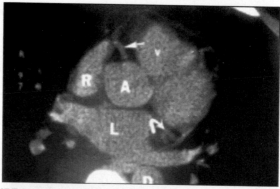

FIGURE 12.4: Origin of the RCA (arrow) The LCX (curved white arrow) is also seen; A = ascending aorta; R = right atrium; V = right ventricle; D = descending aorta—plain CT scan

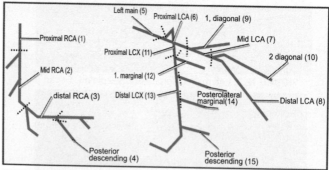

FIGURE 12.5: LAD = left anterior descending artery; LCX = left circumflex artery; LMA = left main coronary artery; PDA = posterior descending artery; RCA = right coronary artery

CONTRAST ENHANCED CORONARY CT SHOWING NORMAL ANATOMY

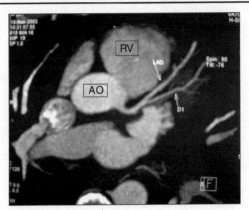

FIGURE 12.6: Coronary CT showing the left anterior descending coronary artery (lad) and diagnol branches

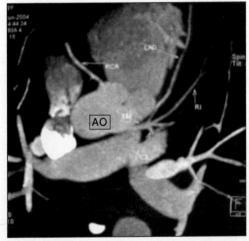

FIGURE 12.7: Coronary CT showing the origin of right coronary (rca), left main coronary artery (lma), left anterior descending

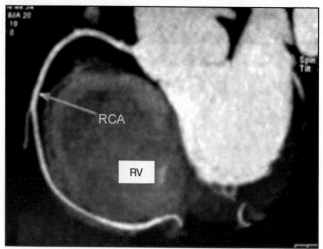

FIGURE 12.8: Coronary CT showing curved refromation of right main coronary artery. RV—Right ventricle

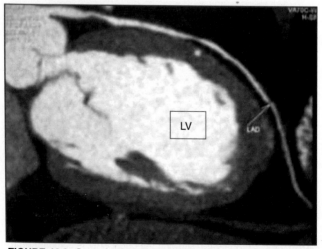

FIGURE 12.9: Curved reformation of left anterior descending artery. LV—Left ventricle

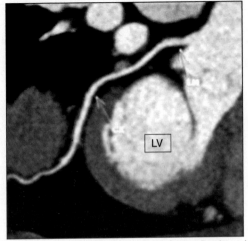

FIGURE 12.10: Curved reformation of the circumflex branch of left coronary. LV—Left ventricle

Index